Fuel
Your
Recovery!

Healing with Nutrition in the Journey from Addiction

Nicole Fetterly, RD, MSc

◆ FriesenPress

One Printers Way
Altona, MB R0G 0B0
Canada

www.friesenpress.com

ISBN
978-1-03-832431-3 (Hardcover)
978-1-03-832430-6 (Paperback)
978-1-03-832432-0 (eBook)

1. HEALTH & FITNESS, NUTRITION

Distributed to the trade by The Ingram Book Company

Table of Contents

Preface

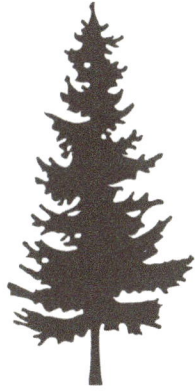

I am a dietitian. I am also an alcoholic. But until I started the journey of recovery, I had never intentionally used nutrition to combat addiction. Addiction and recovery have been key facets of my life for the last 30 years. Although I'd been struggling personally for many years prior, when my only brother took his life after a long battle with addiction and mental health, I really started to spiral. Finally, after 5 years living in regret over his death and my prison of acute addiction and delusion, it was time for me to make the very big change that I had feared more than anything since losing him.

Giving up my substances, alcohol and cannabis, the friends which gave me comfort in my grief and relief from my anxiety, was my only way forward. I haven't looked back since. During my 4 weeks in treatment, I was able to gain clarity, creativity and spirituality that my substances and regret had prevented me from tapping into. I also became aware that my skills, knowledge and experience as a dietitian were sorely lacking in the recovery sphere and it made complete sense to tie the two together in my way to give back and help others suffering with addiction.

Despite my addiction, I have always been very high-functioning and dedicated to my family, friends and my profession. After completing my first degree in anthropology, I realized I wanted a more concrete science background to truly help those I wanted to work with, not just study them. I chose a degree in dietetics that would provide me with a qualification to use immediately upon graduation and I also fell in love with the subject of food, nutrition and health.

I knew I wanted to help clients to make food and nutrition modifications that might prevent them from ending up in the hospital system. I also knew that I wanted to build food literacy and cooking skills with clients, because as dietitians, we can make all the nutrient recommendations needed but if clients do not know how to put these foods on their plate and enjoy them, they will not be successful at meeting these nutrient needs.

I was fortunate to be offered the job of Nutrition Operations Manager at a chain of natural and organic grocery stores in British Columbia. In this role, I developed a love of writing about food and nutrition and co-authored several books for the stores to sell on the topics of gluten-free foods, feeding children and sustainability. We began a cooking program to highlight various foods and their nutrient benefits, that customers could choose and showing them practically how to use them. Of course tasting these delicious foods was key!

After 5 years working in this role, I decided I needed a new audience. The natural and organic customers were already well on their way to optimizing their food choices and I knew there were so many other demographics of people who needed more support and inspiration.

I was offered the opportunity to work at a post-secondary institution as the Manager of Nutrition and Wellbeing. Undergraduate students were the perfect target audience as they are at a time in their lives where they begin to make autonomous food decisions outside of their family homes. I discovered that so many of them had never shopped or cooked for themselves and were prone to living on the typical "college" foods of instant noodles and granola bars. This is not unlike the food that many struggling with addiction rely on when prioritizing their substances over their wellbeing.

In 2018, when my brother died, I decided to distract myself from my grief and regret by pursuing my graduate degree, improving not only myself but others with my research. Although it was a struggle, while working full-time as a busy mom of young children, I pushed through and completed it by the end of 2020. I wanted to research Nudge Theory, essentially an approach of using marketing tactics for public good, not just selling (unhealthy) products. I hoped to influence undergraduate students to make better food choices, like eating more fruits and vegetables.

To increase their knowledge and reach a larger group of people than in one-on-one counselling, I began teaching an undergraduate nutrition course on campus. It fed my soul to share my knowledge of food and nutrition with them in practical and inspiring ways. When they would thank me and share that it was their favourite class or stop me randomly on a hike with my family and gush like I was a celebrity, I knew I had truly touched them with my teaching.

My only regret is the time I spent teaching when I was not fully present due to my addiction and substance abuse, which had ramped up after my brother's death and during the COVID-19 pandemic. Alcohol and cannabis became the priority over my students and although they still learned, I was not as connected and engaged as I could've been. I also felt like a hypocrite when I taught the section on alcohol and how much of a toxin it is in our bodies.

Currently, I work as a Program Manager for a public health program, that works with families to inspire them in their journeys toward healthy living behaviour change. And I am changing alongside them, by increasing my physical activity and improving my own eating while recovering from my addictions. Working as a professional in public health, I feared the stigma of seeking help for my addiction, but I decided I had no other choice but to take time off work to focus on my own wellbeing so that I could truly help others in theirs.

This book is the story of my journey with substance abuse, my fight to escape from the vicious cycle of addiction and the lessons I have learned in recovery, especially regarding the power of food in healing. I hope it provides you or those you love with practical advice and evidence-based learning to embrace food as a key component of a successful recovery, and most importantly, overall well-being.

I dedicate this book to my brother Jesse, who said he was going to treatment for both of us. Although he did not succeed in recovery, I believe my journey honours him and the incredible person he was. My inspiration also comes from my loving family, my husband Paul who has supported me despite all I have put him through with my disease. My wonderful children, Nora and Max, who have kept me going every day to be the amazing mother I have always wanted to be as well as my extended family and friends who have surrounded me with solace, kept me laughing and made me feel so loved. I couldn't have done any of this without all of you.

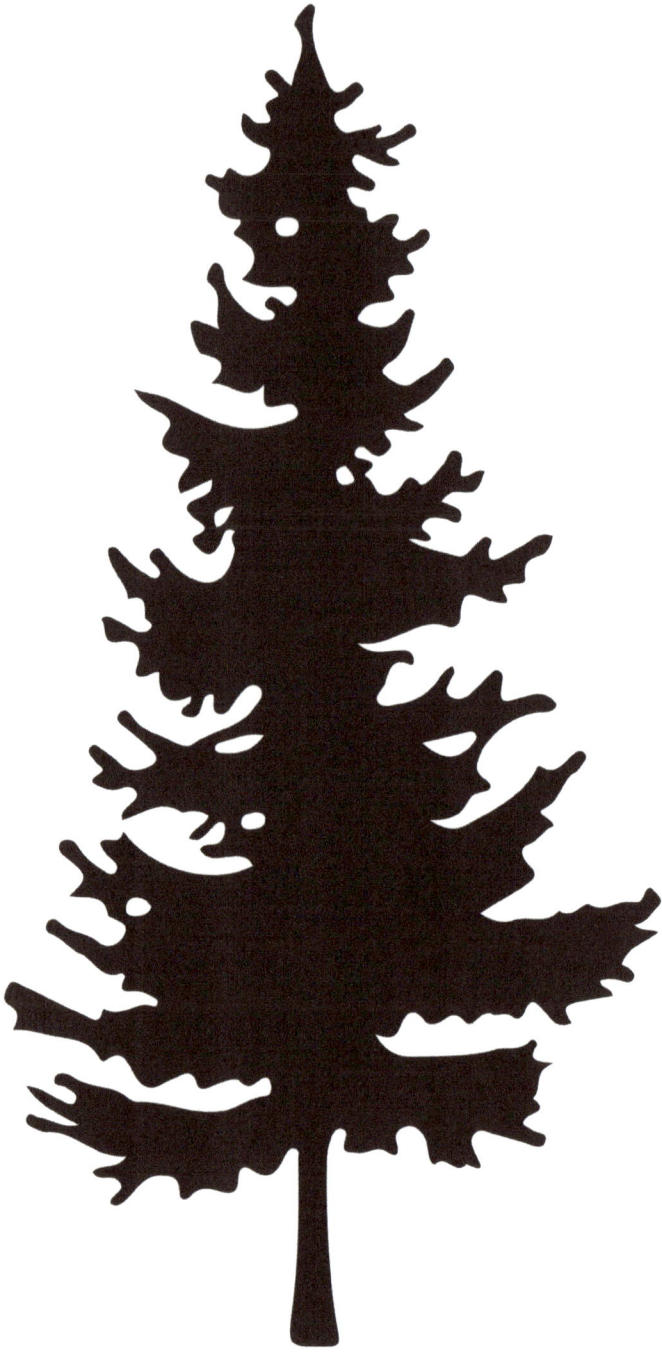

Prayer to the Trees

Please let me root down into the earth, as deep as you grow.

Please let me feel the breezes that blow me, but never let me topple.

Let me collect snow in my branches, but let the
warm, glorious sun melt and free them.

Please let me be the oxygen, in kindness and care, to my family, friends
and strangers, but most importantly myself, to ward off ambition
and restlessness and finally find peace, because I am enough.

Introduction

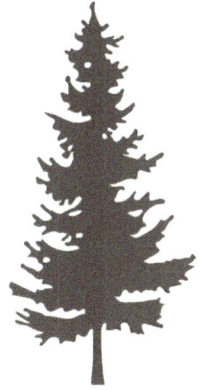

Booze rules…my life, that is. It has soaked into every cell, every thought and certainly most of my actions. I'm a 47 year old woman, mother, wife, dietitian, alcoholic, addict. No it doesn't represent who I am, but it takes up more space in my life than I want it to and it has long been getting in the way of whom I truly want to be.

Booze has been a part of my life since before I can remember. And although I've lost a lot of memories to excess booze, it features into more memories than I can count.

It started as a wee one on my Poppa's knee. There are photos of almost all his grandchildren clutching his lunch beer bottle and as young children do, putting it into their mouth. Of course we were given a sip as we got older and the adults would laugh as we'd grimace at the taste and fizz. As I grew, my grandfather's love of alcohol would feature heavily in my life. I adored my grandparents more than anything and would always spend as much time as I could with them for holidays. For as long as I knew him, my Poppa walked with two canes and had a built-up shoe because of severe juvenile arthritis and one leg being shorter than the other.

His impaired mobility meant, we fetched a lot for him. And the thing we fetched the most was booze. It started with his sherry and cheese at lunch. Then moving onto his beer. He loved to buy "high-test". Back then, it was brands like Wildcat Extreme that had 8% alcohol versus the usual 4% Molson Ex. He was always looking for the most bang for his buck.

Then after his nap (who can have 2 or 3 drinks at lunch and not need one!), he'd come out and be ready for happy hour. In the summer at the cottage, this often involved fancy blender daiquiris with summer fruit or perhaps champagne because of a special occasion. Champs was essential for any function in my family—a birthday, Christmas, weddings or the arrival of someone from faraway. As kids, we helped pass the drinks and got non-alcoholic versions for our own participation and "grooming" in happy hour. By the time we were 15 or so, we got to move onto the real stuff.

At home, it wasn't much different. One of the memories that hasn't been lost is mistaking a glass of my Dad's Scotch one evening for my apple juice. Needless to say, that horrifying sip, not to mention the regular smell of it on my father's breath, left a distaste in my mouth and Scotch became the one spirit I never touched.

My parents divorced when I was 9 years old and I was emotionally neglected, socially anxious as a kid who had been pushed ahead a grade and incredibly fearful. A couple of years later, my mom got remarried. The guy had 3 older teenagers, the youngest being a 15 year old girl, who when I was 11, I idolized. Obviously, she had a leather jacket! And as a product of a "broken home" herself, not to mention having two older brothers, she was a bit ahead of the partying curve.

At the wedding, my new step dad convinced my mom to buy cases of light beer for "the kids". In his defence, his oldest was legal. We spent the whole night in the garage shooting caps and I definitely got my first major buzz. Wow, was I hooked. My social anxiety, especially around older kids (and let me say I was always with older kids because of skipping a grade), dissipated quickly with a couple of drinks. I could laugh and have fun and not be constantly worrying about what everyone thought of me or if I was being too quiet or uncool.

Of course I had to bring this newfound tool and sensation into my life with my friends. It started with a grade 7 party. I was the kid who snuck the Creme de Menthe out of my mom's cupboard. It was pretty much all that was in there—she didn't keep booze in the house. Later she'd say it was because of me but I know she also couldn't leave it alone.

Then there was the party for which I was hired by my mom's friend to be the cute little cocktail waitress. I got caught drinking the dregs of the glasses in the kitchen. As previously mentioned, because I had skipped a grade, I was only 11 years old when this all started in grade 7. Why was an

11 year old drinking booze by herself? Well, that's a question I continually try to answer.

My most significant incident happened in grade 8, at not even 13 years old. I was heading to my friend's cottage with her family for the weekend. She knew some other people in this cottage community and I'd never visited before. Well, meeting people sparked a terror in me so I turned to my new solution…booze!

My dad's house turned out to be my Mecca! He also had a problem but he treated it a little differently from my mom. He valued keeping a very well-stocked liquor cabinet. Perfect! I found a couple of empty pickle jars. I filled one with straight vodka. I filled the other with white rum (when I got caught they thought it was dark rum but I'd actually poured a Coke into it for palatability). I popped them in my duffel and off we went to the cottage.

We made plans to meet up with these skater boys my friend had met before. I was so nervous. It didn't help that my friend was full of confidence, gorgeous and seemed to have no trouble at all talking to people, especially cute boys. I lived in her shadow and to me, booze was my ticket out. A way to show the real me— funny, quirky, with a love of music and dancing, which I only felt comfortable doing after a few drinks.

So we poured a couple of OJs in the kitchen then went into the bunk room and topped up with the vodka. Keep in mind, this was basically our first time drinking the hard stuff. We caught a buzz really quickly. At dinner with her folks, we were hysterical. Everything was funny! Her parents thought we were just silly kids…truthfully we were often pretty hysterical over dumb shit.

We were allowed to go meet these guys and they had picked up some beer. Add that onto what we'd already consumed (and probably little food at dinner with our giggly distractions), and I was shitfaced. My friend said she knew something was wrong when I started hucking empty beer bottles over my head to smash on the ground behind me. Her parents picked us up around 10pm as it got dark and I had to lay my head on the cool glass of the window. That's the last thing I remember of that night, aka my first blackout, at age 12.

These are the gory details that got filled in for me. We were sleeping in the bunk room and I fell off the top bunk. Then I tried the bottom bunk and fell off that too. Obviously the noise was enough to disturb her parents and truthfully she was probably getting a bit worried about me herself. I must've been pretty wasted, as I was suffering my first blackout, so they assumed I had had a concussion and decided they should take me to the emergency room. Luckily (for me, not her parents) I puked all over their Jeep Cherokee the whole way there, so I didn't have to get my stomach pumped. Still the diagnosis was alcohol poisoning and dehydration and for an 80lb 12 year old, that gets you a hospital bed for the night.

My first memory after our car ride home from the skatepark was waking up in a hospital room with three older ladies in the other beds. They were all talking about me. Then I heard the familiar sound of my mom's heels clacking down a hospital corridor. She was a doctor and I'd spent a lot of time in hospitals waiting for her. This time, she was waiting for me to wake up. Was she ever pissed.

I won't get into the details of my punishment. Let's just say I was pretty much grounded from then until I finished high school. My friend and I were told we were "poison" together and they tried to keep us apart but that was futile. We remained friends although she didn't admit to her parents that she was also drinking, which made me appear to be even more of the closet pre-teen alcoholic!

My parents put me into counselling for the first time. I wish they had understood how their unhappy marriage and divorce affected me and had got me help sooner. All I recall is how often the shrink said "street drugs" and how my parents kept asking "why are you doing this to us?".

High school went along in the same way as many teens. Not like for the jocks and the nerds whom I eschewed, but the "normal" teens. I got good grades but started smoking and hanging out in the "pit" next to the cafeteria where I met all the other teen partiers. Weekends revolved around sourcing and drinking booze. We'd spend the first part of the night fishing outside the beer store. Back then a 6 pack among 3 girls was a solid buzz! And that was all our allowance would really let us buy. Of course, my dad's liquor cabinet was extremely well-monitored after that, line markings on the bottles and all.

We drank in fields, ravines, so-called "bush parties" but also often friends' garages or basements where parents turned a blind eye. Flashback to one of those nights where we somehow got a hold of a bottle of Long Island Iced Tea Mix. We were hanging out in my friend's basement. Well after about half that bottle, I was wasted. There was no bathroom in the basement so when I realized I was sick, I had to go up to the main floor of the fancy house and find the powder room, where I puked my guts out. As a wasted 14 year old, I'm sure I did not clean it up well afterwards. And I haven't drunk a Long Island Iced Tea since that night.

Why is it that we can make ourselves so sick on this substance and still go back to it time and again? Even as I write these memoirs, I'm looking back with nostalgia not horror. This is how messed up my relationship with this toxin still is. I love it and hate it, but as they say, addiction is loving something that will never love you back..

The rest of high school went on pretty much the same but add in a few other "fun" substances like hash, weed, mushrooms, LSD, speed, tobacco. But this isn't a book about psychedelics so I won't go into my good (and bad) acid trips or tell you about doing speed for an assembly at school.

All of my arguments with my parents when I got caught for something involved me making my case that I got good grades and was just doing what all of my friends were doing. So life continued on.

Jump ahead to high school graduation, deferring my acceptance to university for a year, and my friend and I taking the trip of a lifetime backpacking around Europe. I was 17 years old, and as my mom said from seeing the pictures, we drank our way through about 10 countries, loving every minute together. Of course Amsterdam was one of my essential destinations and I loved the legal cannabis cafes. As we left for Belgium though, I realized I still had quite the stash and I was scared to cross the border with it. At 6am walking to the train station in the dark, I tried to smoke it all in one fell swoop. I was so high when I got on the train that it felt like we were going to outer space not another country in Europe. And ironically, there was no stop at a border anyway.

When I started at McGill University the next year (which I chose because the drinking age in Quebec is only 18), I quickly found my party peeps. We spent every Thursday, Friday and Saturday night at the Mad Hatter pub, which had the cheapest pitchers in town. I was usually okay if the 3 of us split 3 pitchers, but when I got convinced (easily) to the 4th, plus a few shots, the blackouts came hard and fast. I was lucky that the worst thing that happened was waking up to a guy in my dorm room whose name I didn't know.

The summer after first year, I got a job tree planting in BC and fell in love with the mountains (and a local boy). I decided Quebec was not the place for me and moved to Victoria to finish my anthropology degree. Weed is plentiful out West so my use of it became chronic, every night after school and work, to calm my busy brain and help me sleep.

After university, I travelled to Mexico with the hope of getting to Guatemala, but we ran out of money and ended up getting jobs in Puerto Vallarta and staying there for 3 months. It was an endless party with cheap booze, Mexican brick weed and eventually cocaine, which was very easy to come by. I watched many of my friends become addicted to coke so I mindfully slowed my intake, and stuck with my faves. I also ended up spending a lot more time alone because of it but enjoyed writing in my journal and dreaming about my next chapter of my life.

I came home to Vancouver and got together with my husband-to-be. We moved in to an apartment together in the West End and spent many years of our 20's, back in school at UBC, and partying "normally" with our wonderful friends on weekends. It was the era of raves and ecstasy, which I surprisingly didn't enjoy due to the "drop in" and vomiting. So I stuck with effies (the stimulant ephedrine), which you could legally buy at health food stores, and which allowed me to drink and smoke more without getting tired.

After finishing my second degree, in dietetics, I wanted to fulfill my lifelong dream of motherhood. This is when I started to clue in that my substances, alcohol and cannabis, were hard to give up. I knew I could do it once pregnant, but it was really challenging when we were trying to conceive. After two miscarriages, I finally became pregnant with Nora, and then a couple of years later with Max. Motherhood was tough but I loved pregnancy and being a new parent. Our friends were in the same boat so we were surrounded with fun family times, which still involved a lot of partying. The kids were small so they didn't realize their birthday parties were really just an excuse for me to drink but the timing just changed from staying up all night to raging between 4 and 7pm.

When my son was a toddler, and we were shut out of the Vancouver housing market, we decided to buy a rec property in the Mount Baker foothills in Washington State, next to our friends. This is the period when my day drinking really took off! Everyone would come to visit, camp out and party for the weekend with no worries of driving anywhere. With the booze prices so low across the border, we quickly amassed a huge liquor cabinet. Whiskey in coffee became my breakfast, despite baking lovely treats for my family. I suppressed my appetite and moved into double IPAs before noon and spent the rest of the day maintaining a steady buzz of alcohol and cannabis. This also made me quite lazy so instead of enjoying the natural beauty of the area, the kids and I were happy to putter around the property and laze on the patio.

The cheap booze also started coming home for the weekdays and I was always crafting ways to outsmart the border guards and bring as much as I could. Partially finished boxes of wine were the trick! So then wine became easily available each evening, and socially normalized as the best way to calm busy parenting evenings. But I was still high-functioning, working full-time and advancing my career.

We decided to move to Victoria so we could buy a home and I celebrated my last day of work by sneaking beers in my office and drinking for free at lunch and after work with colleagues. Luckily my friend lent me her bike helmet for the way home because in my intoxicated state, I flew over the handle bars and injured my collarbone. The trip to the hospital revealed nothing was broken but I ended up in a sling and had to shamefully ask my mother-in-law to stay with my husband to do the final pack and clean of our house.

My brother joined us in Victoria a couple of years later and it was clear he was unwell. He sank into psychosis and heavy substance abuse, likely having stopped his bipolar meds. For months, he harassed my family and threatened my husband but I kept in contact, stuck in the middle, knowing he needed help but unclear how to best provide it. Finally after having him arrested, my parents cut him off and he had no choice but to go into treatment. I never saw him again.

The night the police came to our door and told me he was dead from suicide, was the worst of my life. I was already intoxicated but sobered up enough to call my parents who jumped on a plane to come and help. The next morning, I had to tell my kids about their uncle and call my friends and extended family with the news. My best friends jumped on the first ferry and I drowned my sorrows waiting for them. Of course they showed up with cold white wine and in the unseasonably warm weather, we grieved on the sunny deck.

COVID-19 hit a couple of years later and it became easy to hide my drinking while at work or puttering in the garden. I sought support from counsellors and doctors, tried medications, but was unable to stay sober for more than a week at a time. Cannabis was always by my side and I never contemplated giving it up, thinking it was my medicine for sleep and anxiety.

We moved back to Vancouver six years later and I hoped to start a new chapter, but the addiction followed closely. With the stress of the move and trying to find a job, I found myself drinking heavily again and wallowing in regret and shame. I again sought help and found the Daytox program, attending classes, check-ins and acupuncture.

But I kept using for another year. I was no longer able to function without drinking and smoking all day, paralyzed in anxiety when I woke up hungover and desperate to use again. I found isolation in my car, driving to different liquor stores and telling myself I was protecting my family by hiding my consumption in the car.

My kids grew into pre-teens and became well aware I had a problem and didn't hesitate to call me out on being drunk when I was in a rage about the house being messy. My husband quit drinking in revulsion and was struggling to understand my addiction or my grief, becoming angrier. This in turn made me angry, resentful and subversive, but self-harm never has the desired effect of hurting the one you're angry with, unless truthfully that person is yourself.

As a mother, I'm also shocked at how early I used alcohol. I can't fathom my children, at the same age, feeling such need for comfort and self-medication just to cope. Not that they haven't experimented with their friends a bit, as most teens do, but they aren't drawn to it for solace and functioning socially. I am grateful every day that they have so many more tools and a solid foundation to grow into healthy human beings that can hopefully avoid addiction, despite all they have experienced with my substance abuse.

I also sought care from an addiction physician, tried even more medications and learned from her that I had essentially accumulated the equivalent of a royal flush in terms of my risk for addiction. I clearly had the genetic pre-disposition, I had environmental exposure and I had started at such a young age. Although she provided *me* with good care, she was also extremely worried about my kids, and warned me to try to keep them from using so young in life. If I had waited until my later teens or early twenties, my risk would've been significantly less. The only way I can do this is by being open with them about my history and my disease.

After numerous family and friends expressed their concern, I started looking into treatment. My brother's experience weighed heavily, as did the idea of being away from my kids, but I finally knew I had no other choice if I wanted to live to see my children grow up. I was on my way to crashing my car and killing myself or worse, an innocent bystander. Not to mention, my liver and heart health, heightened anxiety and obsession with finding ways to purchase alcohol so my husband couldn't see where I was buying it.

I was so sick, and stuck in this vicious cycle of addiction. I woke up every morning in a state of agony and shame, running through the previous day in my head to determine if I'd exposed my drinking, if I'd left out any of my secret stash. I'd lie in bed, praying to get back to sleep to try to feel better, but it rarely worked. I would make promises to myself that I wouldn't use that day and then remain in a state of brutal anxiety until I gave up my promise. I would always leave at least one drink in the bottle to get me through until the liquor store opened and I would try to hold off consuming it until it was close enough to the time when I could get more. Which I would do every single day, because I didn't "keep any in the house". So 9am would roll around and I'd be back at the store, buying exactly enough for what I needed that day, which of course ratcheted up bit by bit. One 750mL bottle of wine became a 1L bottle, plus 1 or 2 high-test beers to start the morning. I'd given up whiskey a couple of years earlier, because it was too easy to start into in my morning coffee.

I'd hide the recycling, which wasn't difficult living in the city, where friendly people come by to collect and return it. I'd hide the bottles, in various places in the house, and then try to remember where I'd stashed them. I'd hide the cups I had on the go, and be so relieved in the morning when I'd find one I had misplaced, so that I could finish it and know no one else had found it. And through all of this I was deluded enough to think I was getting away with it. The hiding and sneaking, the craftiness, it's all part of the disease and gives part of the dopamine or adrenaline hit that made me feel better.

The final catalyst came with some devastating news that a dear friend, colleague and the doula for both my children, had been diagnosed with stage 4 breast cancer. I knew that if she could spend $30,000 and go away for 4 weeks and come back healed with a new lease on life, she would jump at the chance. I could not let the opportunity pass me by when it had so much potential to change my life.

My nurse practitioner wrote me a note to be off work for 8 weeks and along with my Daytox counsellor helped me overcome the anxiety and shame of taking this time off. I spent 4 weeks in a beautiful treatment centre on Vancouver Island where I gained clarity, creativity and spirituality. Not only did I process the regret over my brother's death and learn about my addiction, but I understood more about my core beliefs ingrained from childhood. Beliefs that I am fearful and powerless had shaped how I processed my brother's death. My belief that I am loyal was challenged as well.

My therapist had me do Cognitive Processing Therapy where I wrote down why I thought he had died and the effects it had on me and my family in the areas of trust, intimacy, esteem and power. She identified my stuck thoughts and with her help and that of my friends in treatment, I was able to reframe these thoughts and free myself and my brother from the prison of my regret.

I found my spirituality in the beautiful forests around the centre and began praying to the trees everyday. I also wrote a lot during treatment—in my journal everyday with the reflections on the important learning I was doing as well as writing poetry, inspired by the sessions with a writer who came to encourage this creative self-expression. Richard's laugh will linger long in my memory—a deep "ha!" that echoed off the high timbered ceiling.

The food at the centre was wonderfully healthy, which meant so much to me as a dietitian. I would start the day with chia pudding, berries and Greek yogurt, topped with hemp hearts which they put out at my request. Lunch was often sandwiches but sometimes nourishing soups that warmed us in the cold weather. Then dinner varied, from chicken to occasionally salmon, with veggies, but when red meat was on the menu, they always prepared me a vegetarian option like tofu or legumes.

The head chef was also a Holistic Nutritionist, which gave him insight into healthy menu planning. However, this qualification does not compare to the education, skills and experience of a Registered Dietitian. He was supposed to offer every client an individual consult but that never occurred while I was in treatment due to holiday staffing shortages.

Instead, other clients would continually ask me questions related to food and nutrition. They wanted support with their digestive health (and chia pudding was my repeated suggestion due to its incredible ability to provide soluble fibre and binding). They also wanted advice on weight management, preventing the common gain that addicts experience when they start eating well again. But for me, as well as some other clients, I lost weight in treatment. This surprised me, as a dietitian, because I knew I had been chronically dehydrated in my addiction and finally consuming adequate fluids (lots of tea!), I thought I would gain water weight. I also struggled to maintain muscle mass due to my excessive alcohol consumption, so I thought I would begin gaining muscle and subsequently weight.

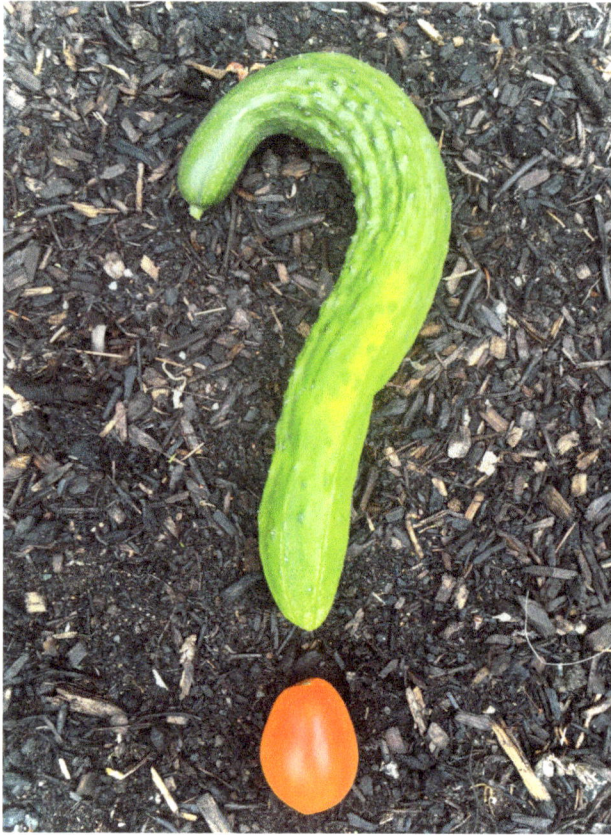

As a dietitian who has founded her practice on providing practical, evidence-based recommendations, I had many ideas take shape about supporting those in recovery. With my clients or students, I focus on which foods to eat, to provide the nutrients they need and support their health goals, and give them strategies to get them on their plates. This may be a different approach than providing a list of nutrients and the amounts needed by a client—I like to say "we eat food, not nutrients".

The last thing I ever share with a client is caloric need—again we don't eat calories, we eat food. Counting calories or other nutrients can take the joy out of eating and can be an inaccurate practice. Although many processed foods are labeled, the foods that should make up the majority of our plates do not have nutrition labels, like vegetables, fruit, whole grains and protein foods.

I believe in the importance of building people's food literacy and their positive relationship with all foods. Cooking at home used to be the norm but that has been lost over the last few decades in North American society, where we now rely on convenience, ultra-processed foods and eating out. It is key to help clients learn how to prepare food for themselves and it does not have to be elaborate meals like we see TV and social media chefs making.

Teaching cooking classes in-person or online has been part of my practice for over a decade and it can be a fantastic way to share nutrition recommendations, build cooking skills and connect with others around a table. I believe this should be an integral component of any addiction treatment centre, but it was not part of the one I attended. Many chefs or administrators may challenge this practice due to safety or staffing restrictions.

However, preparing food does not have to be done in a commercial kitchen, it can happen around a dining table. Ingredients can be laid out for people to build their own overnight oats, chia pudding, meal salads and grain bowls, just to name a few. They can learn to chop and make a meal together, foundational recipes such as soup or curry. By doing this in treatment, clients would connect more deeply to their food and learn skills and recipes they can take home to continue to nourish themselves the way they were nourished in treatment.

Overall my time in treatment was life-changing. The staff and other clients were a constant source of support and the friends I made there will be life-long, people that shared their most vulnerable selves and whom I grew to love in such a short time. My friend, "L", the 70 year old cowboy who lives with chronic pain and yet maintains the sweetest disposition. I knew if he could work so hard at recovery while suffering physically as he did, so could I. My friends "R" and "R" who taught me that I'm not the only one who's lost a brother and we found ways to honour their memories together that didn't involve getting lost in substances. My friend "J", who played beautiful piano, letting me sing along to Stevie Nicks, and DJ'd for New Year's Eve teaching me that my love of dancing, even in front of strangers, was not dependent on having a drink in my hand. These dance parties continued throughout the month with my beautiful friend "M" who helped me not only express my grief in movement, but also in ritual and spirituality. My sweet friend "B" who crocheted scarves for every person at the centre and showed so much strength fighting to regain all she had lost in her addiction. And finally, my new brother "J" who stays in touch better than anyone else and loves me with his whole, beautiful, big, sensitive heart.

I have never stayed anywhere for such a long period that truly began to feel like a home away from home. My room was a haven, where I could escape from conversation (much needed at times) to write, nap or during "tech time" watch a comforting show on my laptop. I also read a lot of books, 1 or 2 a week, which has always been a relaxing activity for me that allows me to focus my brain on someone else's life instead of being in my own head and often unsettled.

I truly hope my story resonates with you wherever you are in your relationship with substances. I want to inspire you, not only with good food and nutrition, but also with my vulnerability and the practical strategies I have used to stay sober and find a new love of life and self.

Please keep reading to learn more about how food, cooking and nutrition can support your body and mind's needs and optimize your wellbeing on your recovery journey. I truly hope you find as much clarity and creativity as I have gained over these last months, as well as use these recommendations to rebuild your strength and heal your body and mind.

At the end of each chapter, you'll find recipes to provide you with nutritious comfort during recovery. The focus should be on whole grains, plant-based proteins, fish, fermented foods and fruit and vegetables. Although poultry and lean red meat can be consumed, most people are well-versed in consuming animal proteins and so for your health and that of our planet, I am providing more plant-based options.

You'll also find summary tips and questions for self-reflection at the end of each chapter, to help you put the readings into practice in a way that works best for you.

Detoxification

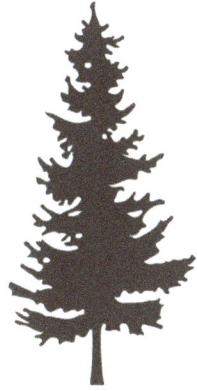

The most well-known stage of addiction recovery is detox. The withdrawal period is different for everyone, lasting from days to weeks, and it should be done under medical supervision. Some of the symptoms of withdrawal can include:

- anxiety
- nausea & vomiting
- headache
- disorientation
- sweating
- agitation
- tremors
- tactile disturbance (e.g. itching)
- auditory or visual disturbances (e.g hearing or seeing things that are not there)

The Clinical Institute Withdrawal Assessment (CIWA) scale should be administered by a health professional regularly to determine the level of withdrawal of the patient and the necessary treatment to manage it (https://www.cmaj.ca/content/cmaj/160/5/675.full.pdf). This treatment could involve medications to manage anxiety and nausea but there are also nutrition remedies that can support you.

When I arrived at the treatment centre, I had been drinking heavily for the days leading up, feeling anxious about my decision to go. I drank the whole way there and arrived with a blood alcohol level of 0.08, not the highest they had seen on arrival! They prescribed some medications to help with my withdrawal symptoms, but I only needed to take them for a couple of days, which they determined by using the CIWA scale above, and by my own reports of how I was feeling. On the first night, I cried myself to sleep, but then over the first quiet weekend, I took time to settle in, rest and start making connections.

This is not the case for everyone. Some people enter treatment in a much more depleted state and need a week or more to detox. They may experience severe vomiting and other symptoms, and some even require hospitalization for IV fluids. Overall, those in withdrawal are heavily monitored, with regular nursing checks, even in treatment centres.

Most people in addiction have been depriving their bodies of key nutrients, like water, energy and vitamins and minerals, either through low intake, malabsorption or vomiting. The major detoxification organs of the body, the liver and kidneys, have been heavily taxed trying to rid the body of the toxic substances that were consumed heavily.

For those withdrawing from chronic alcohol use, there are a number of nutrients to focus on to support the chronic dehydration and malabsorption that has been occurring. Hydrating fluids with electrolytes, like sodium and potassium, are critical to restoring the body's water and pH balance and support the kidney in its metabolic roles.

Water is key but some may find that a homemade electrolyte replacement fluid is more palatable and provides a more absorbable fluid. I like to call this *Nikki-ade* (find the recipe in the chapter *Focus on Fluids*) and it is much more affordable and accessible than the brand name sports drinks, as well as being free of the artificial colouring and other chemicals.

Another key set of nutrients in alcohol withdrawal are the B vitamins. These become chronically low due to malabsorption as well as potential low intake, when alcohol supplants nutritious food.

Thiamine or vitamin B1 is required by the body to metabolize carbohydrates and for proper nerve function. It can be found readily in whole grains, legumes, nuts and meat, although supplementation is recommended for alcohol withdrawal in the range of 250-500 mg/day. To support continued B1 needs, consider soft, easily digestible foods like oatmeal, **Brown Rice Congee** (find the recipe at the end of this chapter), lentil soup or peanut butter on whole grain bread.

The liver has likely been affected by chronic alcohol consumption. A laboratory test is recommended to check the liver enzymes to assess the state of liver damage and to monitor improvement. Many people have liver disease with few symptoms but luckily the organ is highly regenerative. The liver is responsible for more than 500 vital functions in your body, processing everything you eat, drink, breathe or absorb through your skin. The liver regulates your body's fuel and your hormone balance as well as producing essential immune and blood proteins, and cleansing your blood of toxins like alcohol and other drugs.

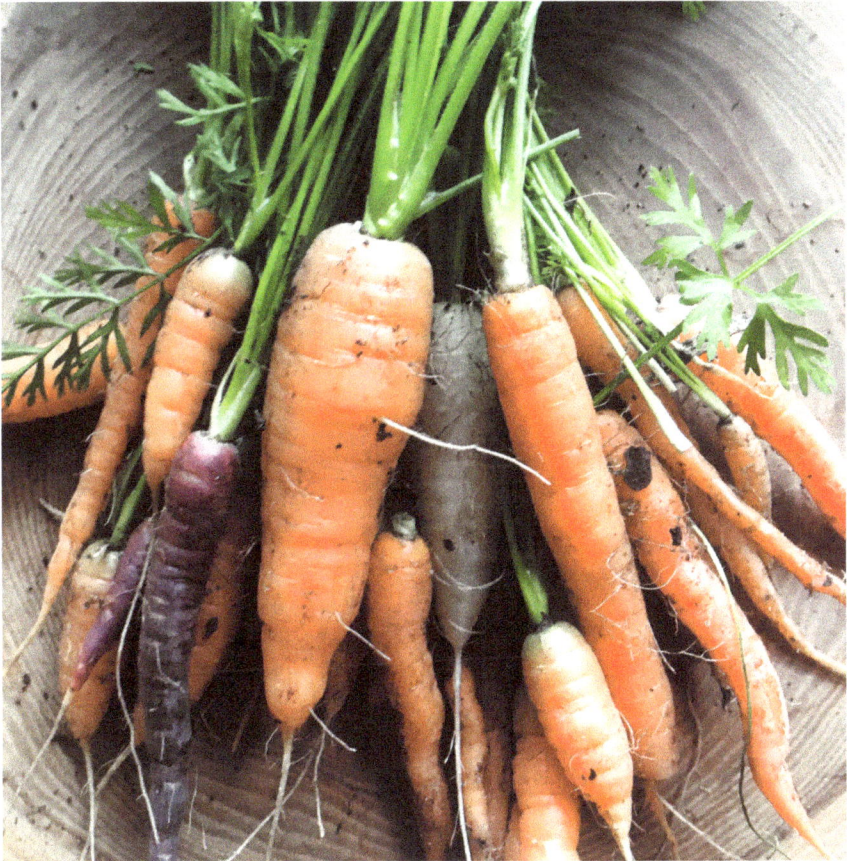

Antioxidants, from colourful fruit and vegetables are key for liver health and so many other immune functions in the body, quenching the free radicals that can cause oxidative damage linked to heart disease and cancer. Aim for half of your plate to be vegetables and fruit at each meal and snack. For some, cooked or pureed may be easier to digest, especially in the early stages of withdrawal as the gut recovers.

Minimizing animal (saturated) fat, from red meat, high-fat dairy and processed foods, and added sugar, especially from beverages, is also key to reduce impact on the liver. Choose plant proteins, like beans, peas and lentils, or fish and use healthy oils, like olive, avocado or canola. See the chapter *Focus on Fluids* for alternatives to sugar-sweetened beverages like soda pop or sweetened coffee and tea. Choose healthier sweet treats, with added protein like the *Chocolate Pudding* recipe at the end of this chapter, or try fruit and yogurt, applesauce or date-sweetened protein balls.

Tips for Detoxing

- Everyone is different—pay attention to the way you are feeling and report any symptoms to your healthcare professionals
- Focus on fluids, especially if vomiting or diarrhea is occurring
- Low appetite and fatigue are common—eat and drink what gives you comfort and don't stress about nutrition at this stage

Self-Reflection

Have a plan in place whether you're detoxing in treatment or at home. Who can you call for support? Who can help monitor you for symptoms of withdrawal?

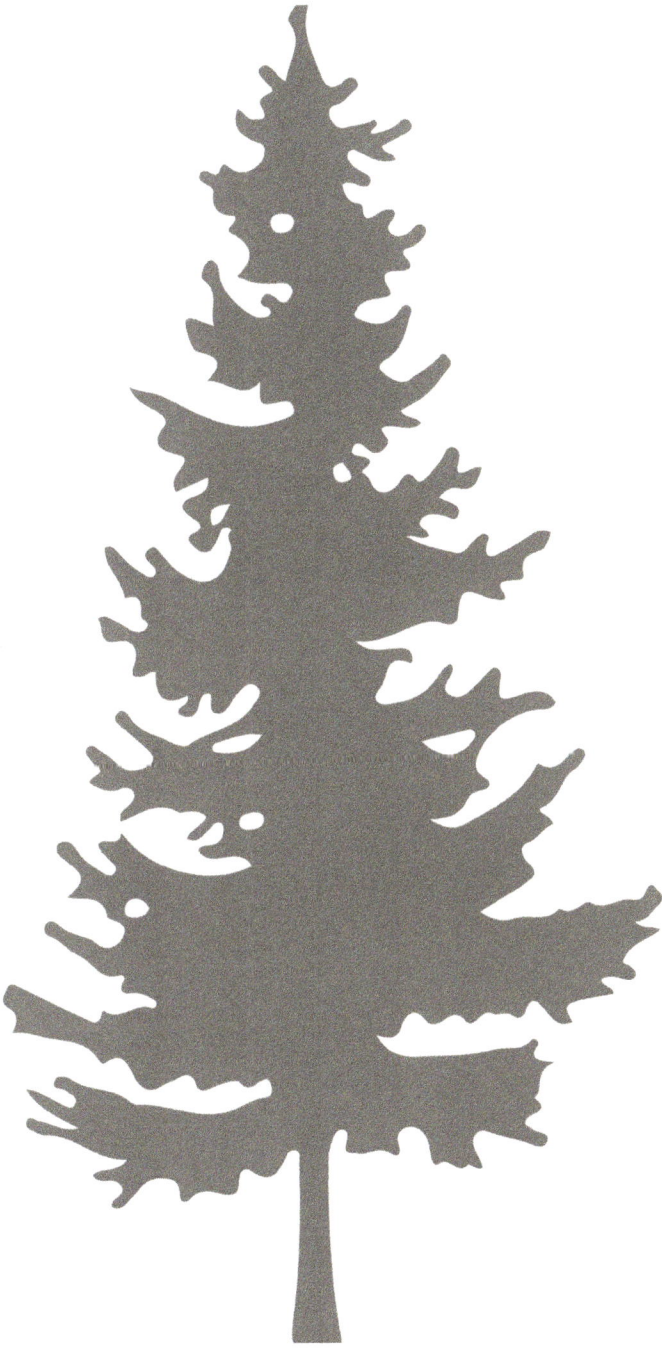

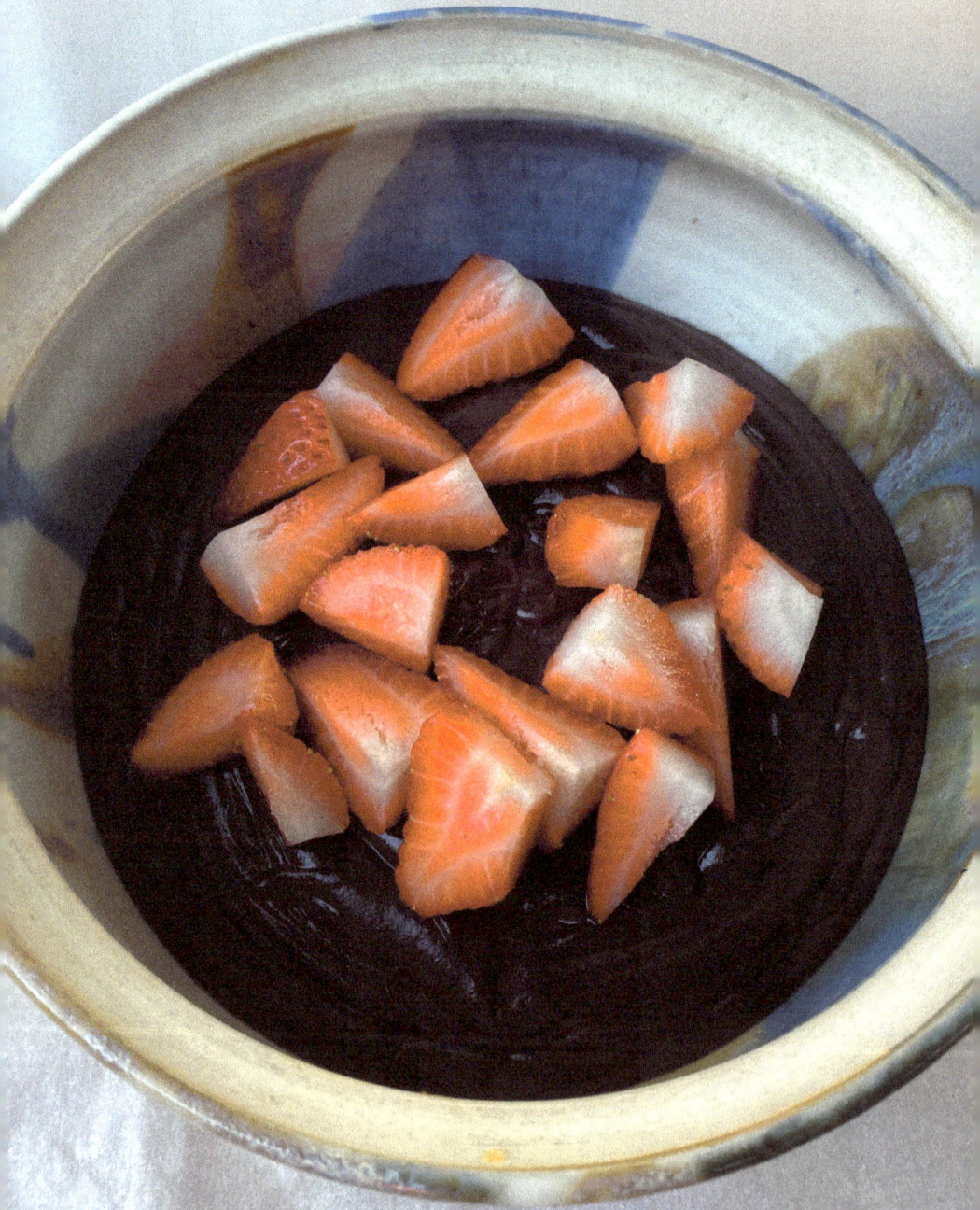

Amy's Chocolate Pudding

The incredible chef that nourished me during my inpatient treatment shared this delicious, easy recipe packed with protein and comfort.

Serves 6

10 hard boiled eggs
1/2 cup dark, unsweetened
cocoa powder
1/2 cup maple syrup

1/2 cup milk
1 tsp vanilla extract
1/2 tsp cinnamon
Pinch salt

Combine all ingredients in a food processor or blender and puree until smooth and creamy. Serve cold and keep refrigerated for up to a week.

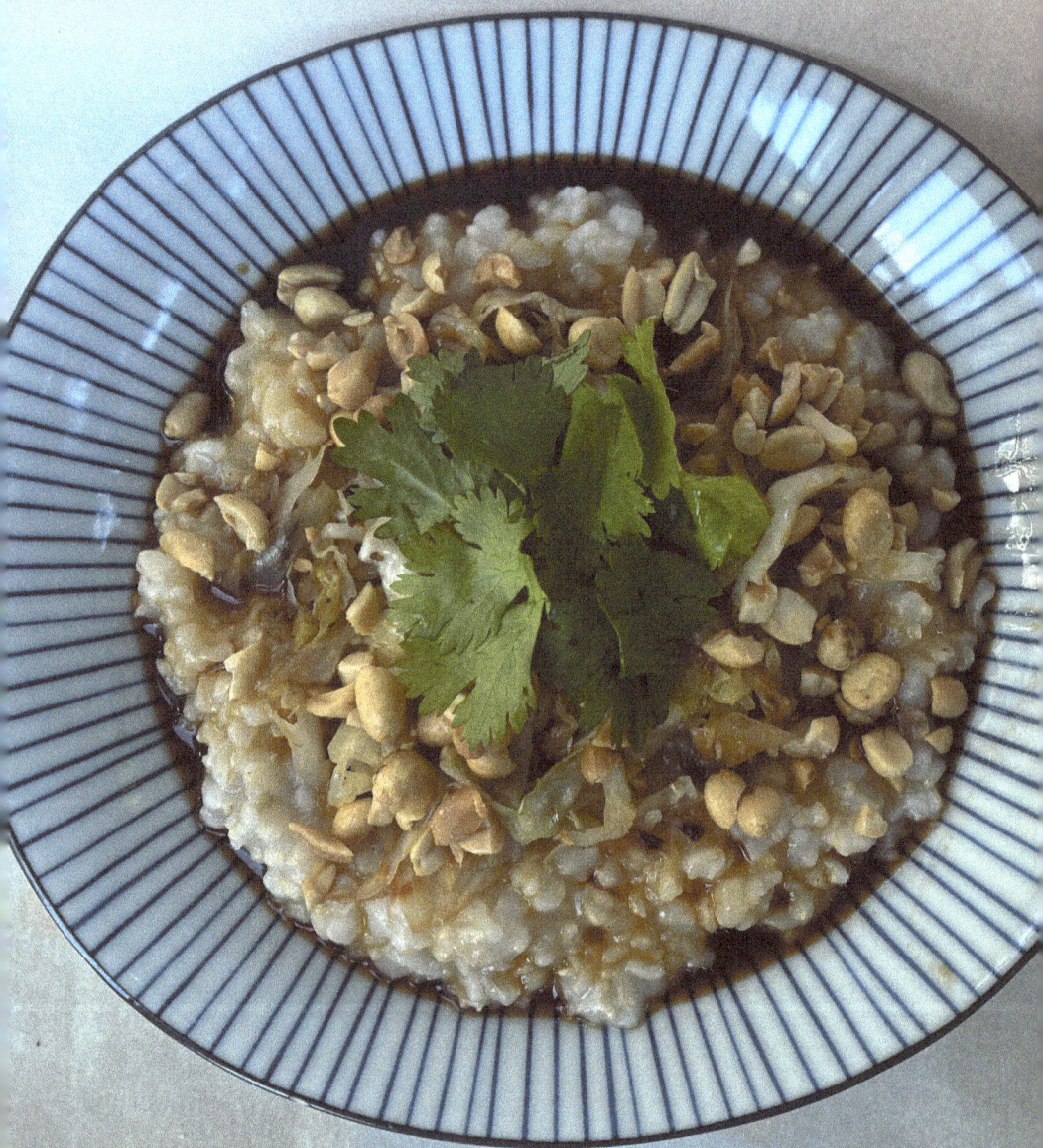

Brown Rice Congee

Congee is a rice porridge consumed in China and other Asian countries for breakfast, lunch or dinner. It can be flavoured with cooked vegetables, cooked fish or meat or chopped peanuts.

Serves 4

2 cups short-grain brown rice
1 tsp salt
10 cups water or vegetable stock
2 Tbsps soy sauce
2 cloves garlic, smashed
1x 1-inch piece ginger, peeled

2 tsp sesame oil
2 tsp apple cider vinegar
Additional cooked vegetables,
fish, meat
Chopped peanuts (optional)

In a large pot, combine rice, salt and water or stock. Bring to a boil then reduce to a simmer and cook until soft and creamy, adding more water or stock to reach desired consistency. Meanwhile, combine the soy sauce, smashed garlic, ginger, sesame oil and vinegar in a jar and allow the flavours to meld. Add cooked vegetables, fish or meat to the rice, if desired, and heat through. Serve hot, garnished with chopped peanuts and a drizzle of the soy sauce mixture.

A Healthy Plate

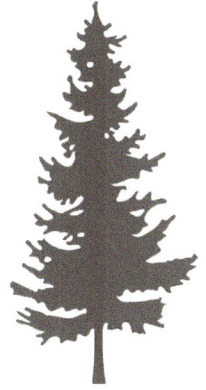

The basis of eating well to nourish your body is to create a balanced plate that is made up of three main food groupings. The first recommendation is for half of your plate at each meal and snack to be made up of vegetables and fruit. Another quarter of your plate can be made up of whole grains or whole grain products, like bread, crackers or noodles. The final quarter of your plate should be made up of protein foods, predominantly plant-based protein foods.

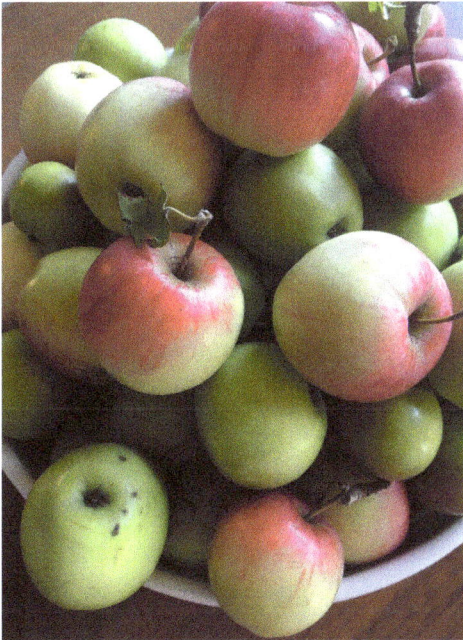

Vegetables and fruit provide us with fibre, vitamins, minerals, other phytonutrients and energy. Veggies and fruit can be consumed fresh, cooked, frozen and thawed or canned and drained. Many believe that cooking, freezing or canning produce can lower the nutrient content but that is not true. When food is frozen or canned, it is often at peak ripeness when nutrients are maximized. Commercial freezing and canning methods preserve these nutrients for us to consume when we eat the food. In fact, fresh produce that travels for long distances from where it is grown and sits on grocery shelves or in our homes, loses nutrients. Frozen and canned vegetables and fruit are also great pantry staples to turn to when you do not have fresh produce, ensuring they still make up half of your plate.

For those struggling with addiction, shopping for fresh foods becomes a low priority, so frozen and canned fruits and vegetables can be available for when there is some time and motivation to eat for wellbeing.

Other ways to optimize fruit and vegetables include making a smoothie, where you can pack in almost half of your day's needs. Add a salad to the side of any lunch or dinner or toss extra veggies, especially those that need to get used up, into soups, casseroles, pastas, stir fries and grain bowls. Cut up fresh vegetables and fruit for easy to access snacks—when we see them, we are more likely to eat them, as opposed to having them packed into a crisper drawer.

However, optimal storage of fresh fruit, vegetables and herbs, is key to minimizing food waste and losing your food budget into the compost. Keep root vegetables, like potatoes, onions, garlic and squash in a dark, cool place like a cupboard or root cellar. Store apples in the refrigerator but separate from other fruit and vegetables as they continue to ripen after picking and produce ethylene gas that causes other produce to ripen more quickly. Store citrus fruits and vegetables like eggplant, peppers and cucumber in your refrigerator produce drawers. For easily damaged or highly perishable items, like greens, berries and mushrooms, wrap them lightly in paper towel to help absorb excess moisture then store in a plastic bag or container that allows some air to enter.

Avocados, tomatoes and bananas should be stored on the counter but they tend to ripen all at once. As soon as avocados are tender at the neck, put them in the refrigerator where they will last another week. Once cut, store them with the pit so they last another day. When you make guacamole, leave the pits in until ready to serve and consider topping with lime juice, which prevents it from turning brown.

When bananas ripen past the point of wanting to eat them raw, toss them whole into the freezer, either in the peel or peeled and in a freezer bag. They can be use to make smoothies or in baking. The same can be done with ripe tomatoes and then they can be used to make soups and sauces.

I was so grateful in treatment that fruits and vegetables were always available, whether thawed berries at breakfast, salad at lunch and dinner or the bowl of fresh fruit on offer at all times.

Whole grains provide our bodies with fibre, energy, B vitamins and key minerals and when grains are refined, much of the fibre, vitamins and minerals are stripped out and only sometimes added back in the process of enrichment. Whole grains include oats, like steel cut, which can be used to make porridge or a "risotto"-like side dish. Rolled oats can be used for overnight oats or muesli, porridge and baking, even grinding them up into oat flour for a finer texture. Brown rice takes longer to cook than white rice so consider making a larger batch, freezing leftovers to add to soups or to make fried rice. Quinoa is a higher protein, higher iron "pseudo-grain" as it is actually a seed. It cooks quickly (15 minutes) and makes a great side dish, grain bowl or meal salad. Cornmeal comes in a variety of textures, from coarse which can be used to make polenta, and finer grinds that can be used in baking and pancakes. Other whole grains, like barley, millet, buckwheat/kasha, amaranth and wheat berries have variable cooking times and flavour profiles. Search for cooking instructions and recipes on the internet or in cook books to try something new like a casserole, soup or summer salad.

Whole grain products include noodles, crackers and breads and they provide much more fibre and other nutrients than their refined grain counterparts. Choose these most often and save refined grain choices for when you are eating out, where it is more rare to find whole grains. For noodles, if whole grain is quite a change from what you are used to, consider the "Smart" varieties that taste like conventional pasta but have added oat fibre to help with digestion and blood sugar. Bread comes in so many options, with one of the best being sprouted grain breads. These are produced with the entire wheat grain intact and sprouted which maximizes nutrients and makes them more digestible. For a softer texture, choose whole grain bread and flatbreads, like roti and tortillas.

Gluten-free grains include rice, quinoa, millet, cornmeal, millet, buckwheat and amaranth. Oats are naturally gluten-free but are often contaminated with wheat in processing and transport. This is only an issue for those with celiac disease (see the chapter on **Dietary Restrictions**), who must strictly avoid gluten, including cross-contamination.

For those without celiac disease or gluten intolerance, there is no need to avoid gluten, which is found in wheat, barley and rye and their derivatives. However in North America, we eat an abundance of wheat, so consider being more grain conscious and if eating wheat at one meal, strive for different grains at other eating opportunities in the day.

In food service, like restaurants and treatment centres, refined grains are the norm and it can help to advocate for whole grain options, like whole grain bread for sandwiches and brown instead of white rice with meals.

Protein foods are key to provide us with the building blocks known as amino acids that form the basis of muscle, neurotransmitters and other key compounds in our body. It is recommended to consume it at almost all meals and snacks as approximately one quarter of your plate. Protein comes from both animal and plant sources. Animal protein foods include chicken, turkey, duck, quail, beef, venison, bison, elk, pork, fish and shellfish, as well as dairy foods like cheese, milk and yogurt. For those that choose to eat animal foods, minimize red, grilled and preserved meats due to their implication in heart disease and cancers, like colon cancer. Poultry and sustainable seafood are better choices for human health and that of our planet. Pork and dairy foods do contain saturated fat, which is implicated in heart health, but they also have a lower impact on climate change than beef.

The best protein choices for our health and the planet, are plant-based protein foods. These include nuts, seeds, beans, peas, lentils and soy foods like tofu, tempeh, soy milk and edamame. Whole grains, like wheat and quinoa, also contain some protein. Aim to include plant-based proteins every day in place of animal foods.

Avoid processed meats, like bacon, salami, pepperoni and hot dogs, which are linked to increased rates of colon cancer and heart disease. For sandwiches and wraps, choose egg or tuna salad or use cooked meats like chicken breast or pulled pork. Or keep them plant-based, with hummus or refried beans.

In treatment, I found the menu was dominated by red meat, which I don't personally eat. They were always prepared to offer me a plant-based alternative (I even coached them on my baked tofu recipe!), but it was not a standard that they included for everyone and I think this is a missed opportunity to introduce a love of legumes. Their rationale was that "people love their meat" and they wanted to provide familiar, comforting foods during a time of so much change. However, legumes are not only the most affordable and sustainable protein on our planet, but they taste delicious when prepared well, and again this is an opportunity to build food literacy and teach people ways to prepare these foods that should be a regular part of our diets.

Overall, with most food choices, I believe in the 80/20 rule. 80 percent of the time, make choices that align with the recommendations in this book (or from other reputable sources like government, educational institutions and non-government organizations). Fill your plate with vegetables and fruit, whole grains and protein foods from plants most often. Then the other 20% of the time, eat other foods that bring you joy or what you have access to, and let go of the guilt associated with food choices for many of us.

Tips to Build a Healthy Plate

- Veggies and fruit should make up half your plate so centre your meal around them
- Add protein, preferably from plant-sources

- Balance your energy with whole grains, like a piece of whole grain toast or crackers

Self-Reflection on Healthy Plates

Avoid striving for perfection. Can you add one extra serving of fruits or veggies to your meal? Can you aim to include two of the food groupings as you get started?

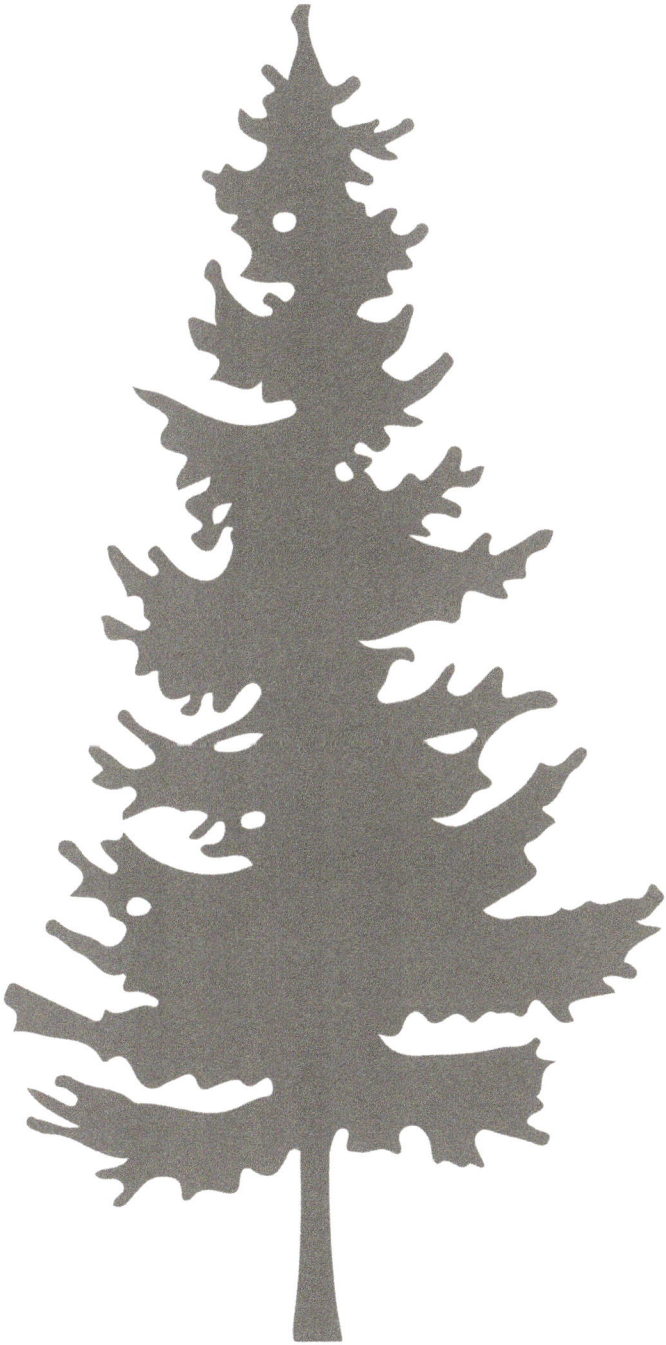

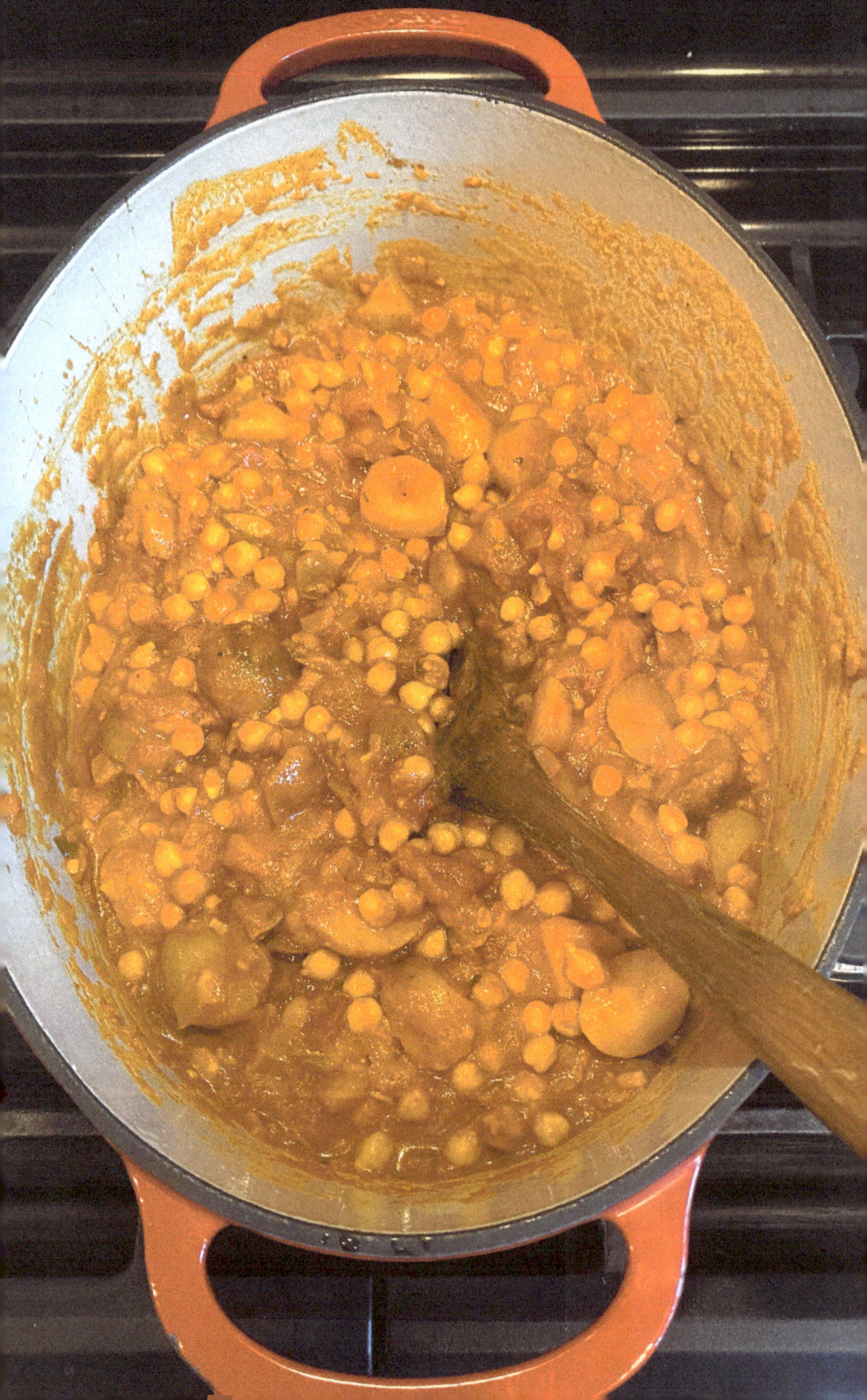

Chickpea Potato Curry

Once you know the basics of curry-making, you can modify it to your preferences of protein, veggies or level of spice. Plant-based proteins are the basis of so much Indian cuisine so curries can be a great way to get these on your plate more often. If you have a food processor, consider pureeing the onion, garlic and ginger to save on chopping but also to form a smoother sauce. The tomatoes can also be pureed.

Serves 6

1/4 cup olive oil

1 onion, chopped

4 cloves garlic, minced

1x 1 inch piece of ginger, minced

3 Tbsp Garam Masala (or your own spice blend—see below)

1 Tbsp turmeric

1 Tbsp salt

1 large can (798 mL) tomatoes, whole or diced

1 can coconut milk

2 cans (398 mL) chickpeas, drained (or substitute chicken)

2 large or 8 nugget potatoes, chopped

Other veggies (e.g. chopped spinach, kale), as desired

Cilantro, chopped (optional)

Hot sauce (optional)

In a large, heavy bottomed pot, heat oil on medium low, then add onion. Saute for 5-10 minutes, until softened, then add garlic and ginger and sauté another 3 minutes. If using pureed onion, garlic and ginger, stir often to prevent sticking. Add spices and salt and saute another 2 minutes. Add tomatoes and cook until the oil glistens on top, approximately 5-10 minutes. This is now called a Masala and is the basis of most curries.

Add the coconut milk and heat until it simmers then add chickpeas and potatoes. Bring back to a simmer then cover partially and stir often to prevent it from sticking. Add small amounts of water as needed. When the potatoes are tender, add any other veggies. At this point, the curry can be kept on low to continue to build flavour or turned off until ready to reheat. Serve with brown rice or whole grain chapati and garnish with fresh cilantro and hot sauce.

Digestive Health And The Microbiome

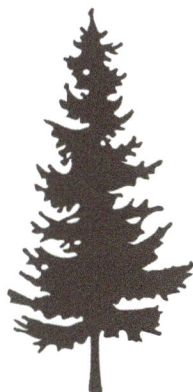

Chronic substance abuse can lead to many complications in the digestive tract, including malabsorption of nutrients and bacterial depletion or imbalance. This can lead to many symptoms, varying in each individual, but can include:

- Mouth ulcers
- Taste alterations
- Dental problems
- Swallowing difficulties
- Acid reflux or heartburn
- Nausea and/or vomiting
- Low appetite
- Stomach ulcers
- Rapid transit (food moving too quickly through the digestive tract)
- Pain and cramping
- Bloating
- Diarrhea
- Constipation

To cope with mouth or dental pain, choose soft foods and nourishing fluids, like smoothies, purees and puddings. For pain and taste changes, consume lots of fluids and consider limiting stronger flavours, like sour or acidic foods and beverages. Eat and drink frequently to ensure adequate nutrition when intake may be limited by pain.

To cope with acid reflux, space liquids 15 minutes before and after eating, to prevent overfilling the stomach. Avoid tightly-fitting clothing and lying down after eating. Avoid coffee, spicy foods and for some, acidic or deep-fried foods, as well as carbonated beverages.

For me, acid reflux does not show up as heartburn, but instead feels like foods are sticking in my chest, especially things like bread or big pieces of meat,. This is actually caused by the lower esophageal sphincter, the valve that prevents food from coming back out of the stomach, becoming inflamed and loose causing the esophagus to go into spasm. Be sure to chew well and try softer foods.

One of my big "aha" moments in treatment, about my potential new path as a dietitian, came from helping a friend with his digestive troubles. On one of our group walks in the nearby forests of Vancouver Island, he shared all of his symptoms and attempts to improve his digestion. I chatted to him about what can improve and deplete our microbiome and gave him some suggestions for what to choose of the food offerings in treatment. A couple of days later, he came running up the stairs in the morning and rushed over to me to say, "I had a great poop! It's working." We jumped up and down in celebration. It's the little things in life that bring us joy, for him a healthy digestive tract and for me, using my knowledge as a dietitian to help others.

Not that everyone in treatment wanted my advice. One of the clients (I won't call this one a friend), was an avid diet-Coke drinker. She chose it first thing in the morning instead of coffee and had the staff stock it for her by the case. After lunch one day, we were all in the gym getting run through a circuit boot camp by the amazing and energetic exercise therapist. This client kept belching, loud guttural burps that she didn't excuse herself for and instead kept blaming the chili we'd eaten for lunch a little earlier. Now I agree that working out right after lunch is not the ideal time, and I also believe in owning our digestive issues and not trying to hold them in, but this was extreme. Everyone else had also had chili for lunch and was not experiencing such obnoxious gas. I happened to mention that it likely wasn't the chili but instead the carbonated beverages she'd consumed heavily. She didn't want to hear it and defended her position vehemently. Sometimes you have to learn to keep your mouth shut, and in this case I mean me, although she could've followed the same advice and kept some of those burps to herself!

Ginger has long been used in traditional medicines for the treatment of nausea and digestive upset. Make a soothing tea by steeping slices of fresh ginger in boiling water, then add honey and/or lemon to taste. Refrigerate leftovers to consume cold or hot as desired. If fresh ginger is not accessible, consider a chewable ginger supplement or a packaged ginger tea. Ginger ales may use real ginger but many commercial varieties do not. They contain considerable added sugar and carbonation which may exacerbate symptoms. Use sparingly.

Other medications are available by prescription or over-the-counter to manage nausea but it is recommended to speak with a health professional as even over-the-counter varieties can have side effects like drowsiness. Proton-pump inhibitors to manage chronic gastro-esophageal reflux disease should only be used under prescription by a health professional and preferably only for a short duration. They work by decreasing the vital stomach acid required to break down foods so chronic use may have implications for digestion and absorption further down the digestive tract.

Vomiting is a more serious side effect of withdrawal as it can lead quickly to dehydration and pose a risk for aspiration or fluid entering the lungs. Consult a health professional if vomiting continues for more than 2-3 days. Ensure fluids and electrolytes are replaced quickly by sipping slowly on "*Nikki-ade*" (see the chapter on **Fluids**) or a purchased electrolyte replacement beverage.

Pain, cramping and bloating are harder symptoms to diagnose as they can have many causes and they differ in each person. Work with a healthcare provider to manage these symptoms and ensure they are not caused by a more severe issue like diverticular disease or ulcers.

Diarrhea can be the result of food moving too quickly through the digestive tract, intolerance to certain foods, excess coffee, medication side effects or bacterial imbalance and other unhealthy organisms. The key is to manage potential dehydration by consuming water and electrolytes. As well, foods that are high in soluble fibre may help with the binding of stool. Try **Chia Pudding** (in the chapter on **Healing Mood with Food**), oatmeal, **Brown Rice Congee** (in the chapter on **Detoxification**) or applesauce. Minimize foods high in insoluble fibre like raw vegetables. For some, an over-the-counter soluble fibre supplement (e.g. psyllium) may help.

Constipation can be caused by low fluid and food intake or as a side effect of many medications. It can also be very uncomfortable and should be managed quickly. Aim for 9-12 cups of fluid per day, including hot water or herbal tea, which can stimulate the movement of the digestive tract, and foods with adequate fibre, like whole grains, fruit and vegetables, legumes, nuts and seeds. Moderate physical activity, like walking, can also help stimulate the digestive tract and help increase appetite.

The Microbiome: Pre and Probiotics

The good bacteria in our gut is a key component of our immune system, digestive health and the regulation of many other functions in our body. It is cultivated from birth, through vaginal delivery, breastfeeding and skin-to-skin contact with our caregivers. These bacteria need prebiotics or fibre to flourish and a diet based on highly processed foods, as well as stress, antibiotics and exposure to unhealthy organisms in unsafe food or water, can throw them out of balance. This imbalance is known as dysbiosis.

The best source of probiotics or good bacteria for humans is fermented foods, but these may be low in the diets of many cultures, especially North Americans. The research is slow to show the benefits of fermented foods as they are harder to quantify in terms of the levels of probiotic bacteria compared to supplements. Choose fermented foods every day, like:

- Plain yogurt
- Plain kefir
- Miso (Japanese soybean paste)
- Tempeh (Indonesian soybean cake)
- Kimchi

- Raw sauerkraut
- Lacto-fermented pickles
- Kombucha
- Sourdough bread

A smoothie can be a fantastic way to pack in fermented dairy foods like plain yogurt or kefir. When dairy is fermented, the bacteria breaks down the lactose sugar, making them more digestible for many individuals. As we age, as well as depending on our ethnic heritage, we may have less ability to digest the lactose sugar in milk. A smoothie can also be a great source of fibre by adding fruit like berries, banana, pear and avocado, veggies like spinach, cucumbers, carrot and plant based protein foods like hemp hearts, ground flax or chia seeds.

Miso paste packs a flavourful punch and loads of nutrients along with probiotics. It can be used as the basis of a dressing or dip like the *Miso Tahini* dressing, which adds more nutrients to salads or veggies than store-bought dressings. It can also be used to make classic miso soup or other soups like ramen, or in sauces, marinades and stir fries. High heat will kill off probiotic bacteria though so use more often in its uncooked form or consider adding the sauce after you have stir fried your vegetables and protein.

Tempeh is a fermented soybean cake that originated in Indonesia. It provides more protein, fibre, iron and other nutrients than tofu because the entire soybean remains intact. It also has more of a meaty texture and flavour. Saute strips of tempeh to add to stir fries, salads or noodle dishes. Alternately, steam tempeh for 10 minutes then cool and crumble. Add spices and soy sauce or salt then form into balls or patties that can be sautéed or baked until crispy. Using sage and thyme, makes these a great plant-based alternative to sausages and for holiday meals.

Kimchi and sauerkraut are traditionally fermented cabbage dishes from Korea and Germany but they can be made with other vegetables as well. Kimchi is spicy, made with chili peppers, and is a delicious topping for a grain or noodle bowl or served alongside dumplings. Sauerkraut is traditionally used to top burgers and sandwiches but is also a great addition to coleslaw. Be sure to choose raw sauerkraut from the refrigerator section of the grocery store as the shelf-stable varieties have been pasteurized which kills off the probiotic bacteria.

Lacto-fermented pickles gain their tartness from fermentation by the Lactobacillus organism, as opposed to vinegar pickles. This means they contain probiotic bacteria if they are stored refrigerated as opposed to being pasteurized or canned like vinegar pickles. Use them on sandwiches, in wraps, with cheese and whole grain crackers or on a veggie platter.

Kombucha is a fermented tea that has gained wild popularity over the last decade. It comes in a wide variety of flavours and with varying levels of sugar. The probiotic bacteria consume the sugar in the fermentation process but then juice is added in a second stage which can add some natural sugar back into the beverage.

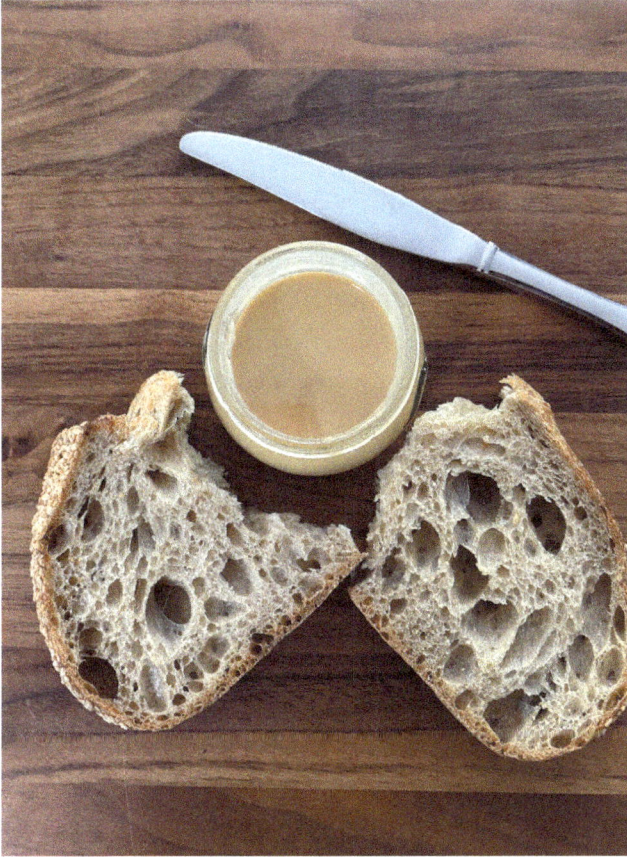

Sourdough bread is fermented but the baking process kills off the probiotic bacteria. So although it is not a source of probiotics, the fermentation of the wheat makes it more digestible for some individuals and it tastes delicious! Choose whole grain sourdough bread for your toast and sandwiches.

For some individuals, a probiotic supplement may be warranted to give the digestive tract a boost of good bacteria. Each brand of supplement provides a slightly different kind or assortment of bacteria and everyone has different needs. Work with a healthcare professional, like a Registered Dietitian, to determine which supplement might be right for you. If you experience more bloating, consider a different strain of bacteria.

As mentioned, probiotic bacteria need prebiotic fibre to flourish. Diets based on highly processed foods are generally very low in fibre whereas cooking at home and focusing on mostly plant foods, can easily provide optimum fibre at the recommended intake level of 30-35 grams per day. Aim for half of your plate to be vegetables or fruit at each meal and snack. Choose plant-based protein foods more often, like beans, peas and lentils, as well as nuts and seeds.

Whole grains are another good source of fibre for our digestive tract so choose them more often than refined grain processed foods like bread, crackers and pasta. Whole grains contain more protein, fat, vitamins and minerals than refined grains, which are often stripped of nutrients when they are prioritized for their starches. Processed food manufacturers will then add some of these nutrients back to enrich the foods with iron and B vitamins, some of which are required by law to manage the nutrient deficiencies that have resulted from overconsumption of refined grains.

Whole grains can be stored in the refrigerator or freezer to protect the fats in them from rancidity and help them last for a long time. They make wonderful pantry staples and can form the basis of meals or side dishes. For grains that need longer to cook, consider making them in large batches and freezing leftovers. For example, make a big batch of brown rice, use what you need for a meal, then store the rest and use for a fried rice dish or to add to a stew or vegetable fritter.

Choose whole grain processed foods more often, like whole or sprouted grain breads which have significantly more fibre and protein than refined grain breads.

Tips for the Microbiome

- Include a fermented food or beverage every day
- Feed the good bacteria with the fibre they desire from whole grains, fruit and veggies, plant-based proteins
- Track your digestive symptoms and seek support from healthcare professionals

Self-reflection on your microbiome

Get up close and personal with your poop. Are you straining to have a bowel movement? Add more fluids, even just hot water, and activity to your day. Are you experiencing loose or watery stools? Add more soluble fibre, like oatmeal or chia seeds.

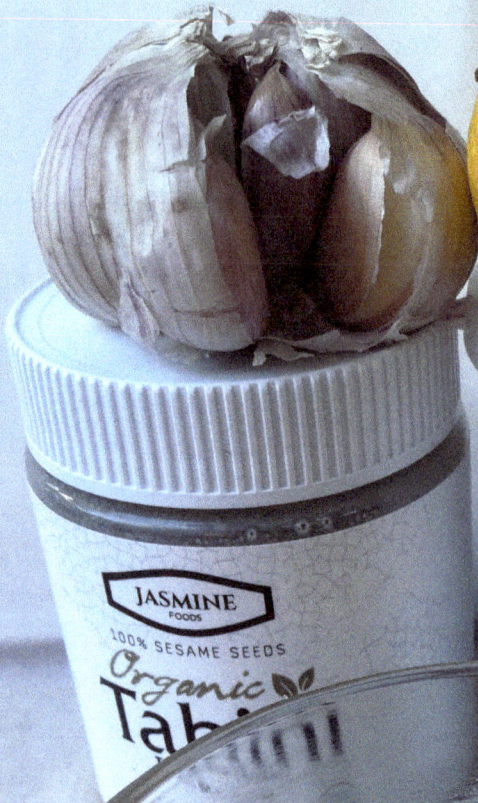

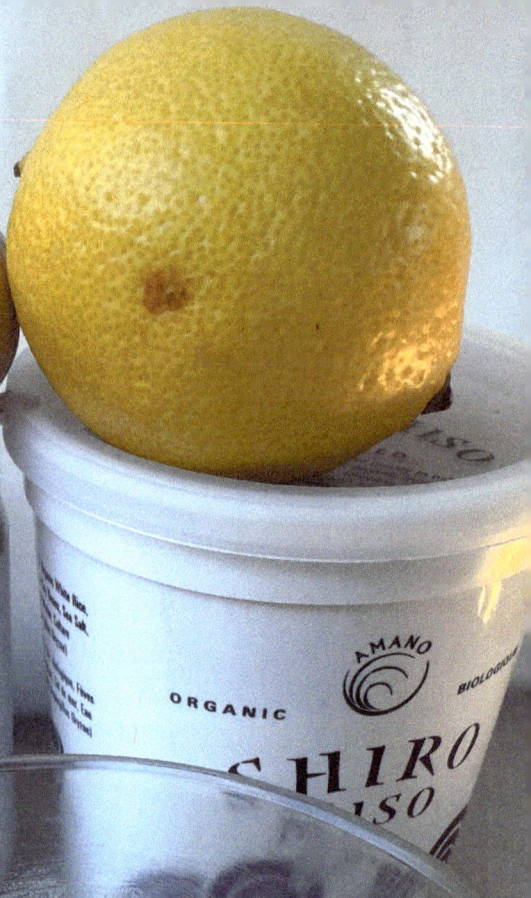

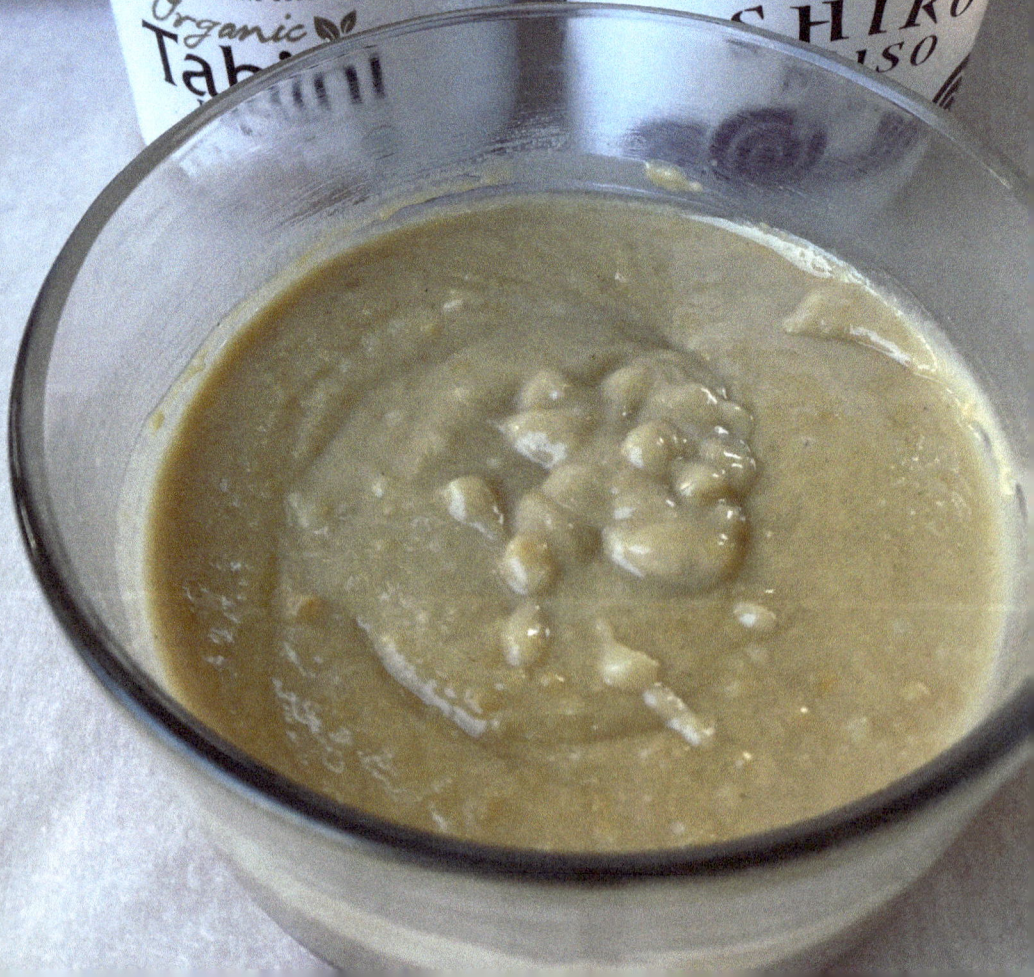

Miso Tahini Sauce

Miso paste is a fermented food from Japan that is packed with nutrients. When paired with tahini or sesame paste, it can make a flavourful, nutritious dip or dressing for vegetables or grain bowls that is easy to make and a better choice than many store-bought salad dressings.

Serves 4

1/4 cup miso paste
1/4 cup tahini
Juice of 1 lemon

2 cloves garlic, minced or pressed
Boiling water to thin

Combine miso, tahini, lemon and garlic in a small bowl then thin to desired consistency with boiling water. Store in the refrigerator for up to a week.

Addiction And Appetite

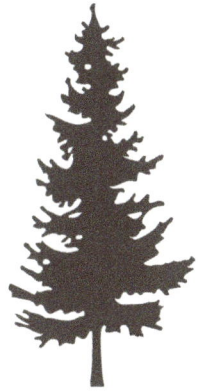

Substance abuse wreaks havoc on the body and mind, altering our hormones and their regulation of hunger. The length of time since the last meal or snack, as well as environmental triggers like the sight, smell or sound of food, can stimulate hunger response in the body and the release of hormones and digestive juices (e.g. our mouth watering) and the classic tummy rumble. In our addiction, however, many of us, mistook these hunger cues for cravings for our substances and consumed those instead of nourishing food. This confuses the brain and makes it more and more difficult to respond properly to hunger.

Other substances, like opiates and stimulants, can decrease appetite and hunger and allow us to function energetically without the critical fuel our body truly needs.

Appetite is not the same as hunger. It can be driven by states of mind, like sadness, stress or boredom. It can be stimulated by environmental triggers even when we are not hungry, like the smell of a freshly baked pie after a large holiday meal or the French fries wafting out of the fast food establishment.

Appetite may make us choose foods that do not ideally support our nutrition needs. It may cause us to replace our substances with food or beverages, for comfort or solace, and for many in early recovery to gain unwanted weight.

For low appetite, make every sip or bite count and try to eat or drink something frequently. Smoothies and other nourishing fluids, like juice or milk, may be easier to consume than food. Some people experiencing nausea and low appetite may find cold foods easier to tolerate as they have less smell than hot foods. Most importantly, consume what is comforting and palatable as any food is better than no food.

My brother and I both struggled with low appetite, especially in the morning. Pressuring people to eat can often backfire as the anxiety that accompanies it, can make appetite worse. Hunger can also be confused with cravings in addiction, when users rely on alcohol and other substances, like cannabis, to calm the stomach.

I had used cannabis for years as an appetite stimulant and I had a hard time eating without it. I had also messed with my body's hunger mechanism, by continually drinking alcohol when hungry instead of eating food, so I had to be cautious, especially in the morning, with coffee. I tried to put the recommendation that I have often given clients who struggle with appetite into practice by limiting myself to 1 or 2 cups of coffee and then making myself eat breakfast before having any more cups.

In treatment, my other appetite issue came around dinnertime. The food was laid out at 5pm, which I found early in terms of being ready to eat. It also coincided with when we were allowed to use our phones, "tech time", and I was usually so excited to speak with my family and friends that I would prioritize that instead of eating. This delayed my dinner until 7pm which meant I wasn't hungry when the evening snack was put out around 9pm and would've given me another opportunity to eat. The snack was usually cheese and fruit, which is great before bed for me, with protein and fibre to fill me up all night.

Some of the evenings, we would also have an additional session—Breathwork or Poetry—and it's hard to eat dinner when you're breathing deeply. This would delay my dinner even more and despite feeling hunger sensations in my body, I would drink tea instead. When we don't respond to our body's hunger cues, it confuses us and can lead to patterns of not eating, just like when I was drinking alcohol excessively.

Pay attention to what your body is telling you and avoid appetite depressants like coffee and nicotine. One strategy might be to delay consuming coffee in the morning or having a cigarette until after eating or drinking something more nutritious. It does not have to be a big breakfast, perhaps just a snack like a fruit and cheese or peanut butter on whole grain toast.

For excess appetite, try to pay attention to the feelings you have that are driving your desire for food and drinks. If it's truly hunger and your tummy is rumbling, then eat something nutritious. If it's the feeling of boredom, try other soothing distractions like having a hot bath, drinking tea, reading a book, writing in your journal, doing some light activity or stretching, meditating, listening to music or a podcast, or phoning a friend.

If it's the feeling of sadness, again reach out for support rather than eat in isolation. Consider making a cooking date with a friend or family member. Choose a recipe or two together and make extra for the freezer.

Some weight gain in early recovery is very natural. Many of us in our addiction were chronically dehydrated and our body is restoring fluid balance. We also may have been undernourished and depleted, unable to maintain muscle mass. When we start eating again, our body may be focused on storage to face the potential of another bout of undernutrition.

Avoid stepping on a scale every day. Once a week is the most often you should check in as our weight can fluctuate daily due to water balance. Instead of fixating on the number on a scale, pay attention to other health metrics, like your waist circumference or whether your clothes are fitting differently. Gaining fat around the waistline is associated with health risk for metabolic syndrome and heart disease as this type of visceral fat surrounds our organs, as opposed to the subcutaneous (under the skin) fat that is important for protection and warmth.

As our activity may increase in recovery, so can our appetite. Be sure to hydrate properly with 9-12 cups of fluid per day and avoid or limit sugar-sweetened beverages like soda or coffee drinks that contain few nutrients.

Mindful eating involves taking the time to eat free of distractions like screens. It involves appreciating each bite of food, paying attention to the senses like how the food looks, smells, feels, sounds and tastes. When we eat mindfully, we can tune into our emotions around eating as well as our hunger and fullness cues. Studies show that areas in the world, like Okinawa, that are known for the longevity of their inhabitants, have mindful eating practices like eating with others, where we can talk and enjoy each other's company. As well, Okinawans tend to eat only until they are 80% full, by eating slowly, instead of rushing to finish and having a second helping before your body can register that it has taken in enough.

Don't feel the need to finish your plate, as many of us were taught in childhood. Many portions, especially those served in restaurants or by others, are more than we are hungry for. Instead, if you're served a large portion, set some aside as leftovers, freezing them if you don't like to eat the same thing the next day. Plus that way, you might save room for dessert!

For some, the pressure or battles they experienced around food may be very triggering. Especially when it comes to finishing the plate or certain types of foods, especially vegetables. My dad would not let us leave the table until we were finished and for me, this struggle was especially apparent with green veggies, like peas. My family would all leave the table and head to the tv room to watch a favourite show. I was left sitting alone staring at a plate of peas. My only option, without having a family dog to eat them, was to swallow my peas whole with a glass of milk or water. This certainly did not give me an appreciation for or a positive relationship with peas to this day.

With my children though, I kept this dislike to myself. Whether consciously or unconsciously, we can influence our children's food choices by sharing our own opinions of what we like or dislike or what we deem healthy or unhealthy. Offer foods to children and adults alike in a neutral way without pressure about the order in which they are eaten and opinions on whether they are tasty or healthy.

Obsession with food can result when we become fixated on our health and that of our food choices. It can become so severe that disordered eating, called Orthorexia, develops where obsession with eating very "clean", healthy food can get in the way of enjoying food, especially with others. Although this book talks a lot about choosing healthy foods more often, all foods fit in a balanced diet and one of the most important parts about food is finding joy in eating all types, especially those from our cultural and family traditions.

Obsession with food can also become a new addiction for those giving up other substances. It can show up in ways like eating in secret, often the way we hid our substance abuse. It can also result in a lot of guilt or shame about our food choices or the quantities we eat of them, which is not representative of a positive relationship with food. Try to avoid feeling guilty about certain food you enjoy, like sugary treats, salty snacks or even cheese, which is highly nutritious and packed with protein and calcium.

Instead strive for an 80:20 approach where the majority of the time you aim for half your plate to be vegetables and fruit with whole grain foods and plant-based protein foods making up the other half. If you eat out only once a week or so, enjoy it and get the French fries or the dessert!.

Tips for appetite

- Be mindful of why you are eating or not eating and try to address the underlying causes
- For low appetite, choose nutrient-dense fluids, like smoothies or milk, over coffee, pop or water and eat or drink every 1-2 hours
- For excess appetite, try to find comfort in other things like getting out in nature, having a hot bath, phoning a friend or drinking a tea

Self reflection on your appetite

We eat for many different reasons. Can you tune into your body's hunger and fullness cues, eating without distractions like screens? Can you take time to savour the preparation and consumption of your foods, noticing how they look, smell, feel and taste?

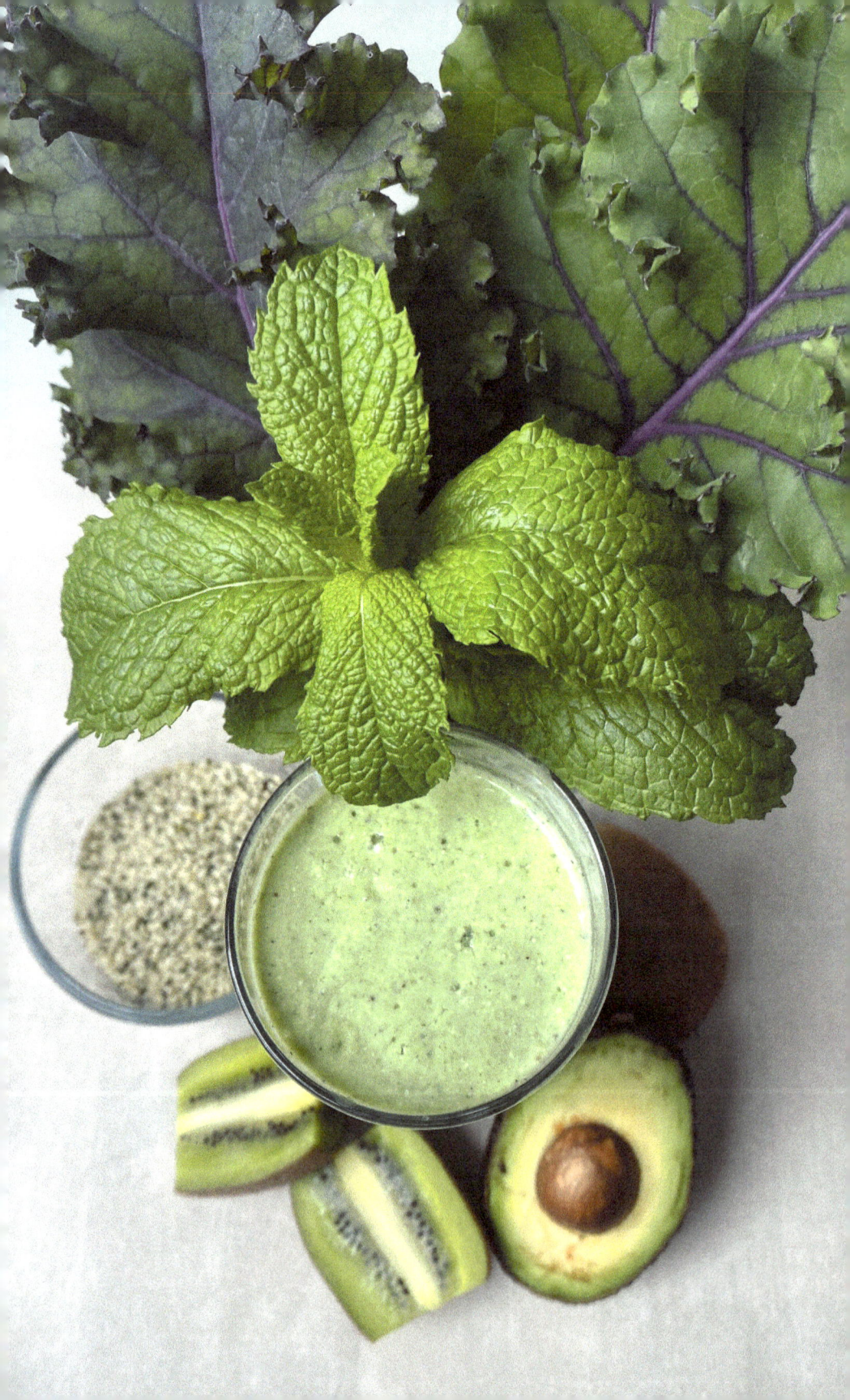

Green Smoothie

A smoothie can be a great way to achieve nourishment when appetite is low or time is tight. Pack in protein and half a day's worth of veggies or fruit in a few gulps. The key for a beautiful bright green colour is to use only light coloured fruit, not dark berries.

Serves 2

1 avocado, pitted and peeled
1 cup dark leafy greens (e.g. spinach, kale)
1 cup plain kefir or yogurt
3 Tbsp hemp hearts

1 pear, cored or other light-coloured fruit (e.g. pineapple, melon, kiwi)
1/2 cup liquid (e.g. milk, orange/ pineapple juice)
1 cup ice

Combine all ingredients in a blender and puree until smooth. Serve immediately.

Healing Mood With Food

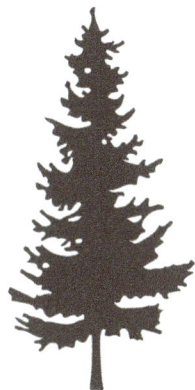

Depression and anxiety are very common concurrent disorders that accompany addiction. When we remove our comforting substances, these disorders may be exacerbated but there are many nutrients that can help support their management.

One of the key tools is to get adequate sleep, which can be a struggle for those in addiction and withdrawal. Limit caffeine, especially after noon. Choose better bedtime snacks, that contain protein and fibre, to help sustain you through the night. A bowl of yogurt with fruit, peanut butter on whole grain toast, a high-fibre cereal with milk or cheese and whole grain crackers or fruit can be good alternatives to sweet treats.

A fruit and cheese platter was commonly served around 9pm in the treatment centre I attended. Not only was it good food to consume before bedtime, but it was a time that we all gathered around in the dining space to discuss the teachings or occurrences of the day. It helps to get these thoughts out of your head so they are not circling around preventing you from falling asleep. If sharing with others is not comfortable, consider writing these thoughts and feelings down in a journal before bed.

As well, focus on building a positive sleep routine by turning off screens an hour beforehand, striving for a regular schedule, going to bed and waking at the same time each day. Other relaxation methods can also help induce sleep, like having a hot bath, meditating, reading a book, drinking herbal tea or doing some breath work.

Protein is key to supporting the brain and providing the building blocks for the chemical messengers, or neurotransmitters, that help our mood. Serotonin is the neurotransmitter that helps you have a more restful sleep and establish your body's internal clock. It also helps us with feelings of wellbeing and happiness. Oxytocin is known as the "love" or "cuddle" chemical that is linked to breastfeeding but in adults, both male and female, helps us build strong connections of loyalty and trust.

Dopamine is the neurotransmitter that helps with wakefulness and coordinated voluntary movements, like writing or driving. It's part of the brain's reward system and many of us in addiction overproduce dopamine from the acquisition or use of our substances. This gives us temporary pleasure or "a high" but we also crash down dramatically after, leading to fatigue, depression and loss of interest in activities. The misuse of substances also confuses the reward pathways in the brain which should normally be activated from survival necessities like food and belonging.

To meet protein needs, consume protein at all meals and snacks. Include plant-based protein foods more than animal ones, like eating peanut butter, nuts and seeds and beans, peas and lentils. Eggs and seafood are also good sources of protein with fatty fish, like salmon also providing essential omega-3 fats that are important for our brain health and immune system.

Healthy fats, like omega 3 mentioned above, are important for mood and brain health, including our cognitive functioning, emotions, behaviours, hormonal and neuronal pathways. They can help us preserve memory, which may have been damaged with substance abuse, and reduce the risk of diseases like Alzheimers. Consuming insufficient healthy fat in our diet (e.g. low-fat diets) can have negative effects on our mood and by consuming enough healthy fats we can lower our risk for depression, which can be so common in addiction and recovery. We should aim to include approximately 30% of our caloric intake from healthy fat foods.

Healthy fats come from fish and plant foods, like olives, nuts and seeds. Use olive oil as your primary added fat, whether in dressings, baking or cooking. Olive oil is one of the key facets of the Mediterranean diet that is known to improve heart health and reduce risk of chronic disease, including Alzheimers. If olive oil is beyond reach of your budget, more affordable plant oils include grapeseed, canola, peanut and avocado. Due to their refinement, these oils can also tolerate higher heat cooking, although generally speaking it is better to cook food slower and at lower temperatures. High heat cooking, deep-frying and grilling, can produce carcinogenic compounds so opt instead for braising, stewing and sautéing on low to medium heat.

Animal fats can contain much higher levels of saturated fats, which are linked to heart disease risk and may not have the benefits of enhancing mood. One of the most common questions I get as a dietitian is "which is better, butter or margarine?". Although butter is an animal fat and therefore saturated, it is also much more natural, with only 1 or 2 ingredients. I like to explain it that you can make butter at home, using cream and a lot of elbow grease, churning it. Margarine on the other hand, although made from plant oils, is not something you can make at home. It is an ultra-processed food-like substance, made mostly from soybean oil, despite the packages claiming better ingredients like olive oil or omega 3.

So my recommendation is to choose butter over margarine but use it in moderation. For example, rather than cook in butter, use olive oil, and save the butter to spread on your toast. Or even better, put something with more nutrients on your toast like avocado or nut butter!

For oils, the 80/20 rule, mentioned in the **Healthy Plate** chapter, would apply by using healthy oil choices like olive and avocado most often. Then the other 20 percent of the time, use butter, ghee, coconut oil, lard or more refined plant-derived oils like canola, grapeseed and peanut.

Essential omega fats are the most important ones to focus on in your food choices because the term "essential" means they cannot be made by the body from other fats. The essential fats are omega 3, 6 and 9 but omega 6 and 9 are much more plentiful in the food supply. Omega 6 is abundant in oils like grapeseed, soy and corn oils. With ultra-processed foods primarily being made with inexpensive oils like soy and corn, if we consume a lot of these foods, we consume a lot of omega 6.

Omega 3 is much less plentiful in the food supply. The sources are predominantly fatty fish, like salmon, trout, herring and sardines, as well as some nuts and seeds, especially ground flax and chia. The recommendation is to include fatty fish at least twice per week but fresh versions can be very costly. Canned salmon and sardines are much more affordable and are fantastic pantry staples to make a meal come together quickly (see the chapter on **Sustainability** for some tasty *Salmon Patties*).

For those who do not consume fatty fish, it is key to include omega-3 rich seeds regularly. Add ground flax, which is the most affordable, to yogurt, smoothies, cereal and baking. The flax seeds must be ground, not whole, for our bodies to access the fats as we cannot break down the tough husk. You can buy them whole and grind them yourself in the blender. It is recommended to store these in the fridge or freezer to protect these essential fats which are easily degraded by light and heat, making them rancid.

Find the recipe at the end of this chapter for *Chia Pudding*, a perfect breakfast or snack, that can be adapted to your tastes or what you have access to, like the type of fruit you add or the liquid you use. Chia (and ground flax) have high quantities of soluble fibre and when they are soaked in liquid, they swell and become gelatinous, making a pudding-type consistency. If this texture is not appealing to you, simply add chia into smoothies, yogurt, hot cereal or baking.

Every morning, in the treatment centre, they offered chia pudding in cute little glass jars and I topped it with thawed berries and Greek yogurt. They even put out hemp hearts at my request. That healthy breakfast has continued for me at home and I have chia pudding in the fridge always ready to go. As other clients saw me eating it and asked me what it was, the staff had to start making more and more, as the little jars became sought after.

Chia and ground flax can also be used to make an egg-free binder that can work in baking. Simply combine 1 Tbsp of the seed with 3 Tbsp of water and allow it to soak for several minutes. This can replace one egg in a baking recipe and then boosts the food's fibre and omega 3 content.

Folate, one of the B vitamins, is also essential in the brain to produce neurotransmitters. It has been linked to improvement of depressive symptoms and memory, both of which can be heavily affected by substance abuse. Folate is plentiful in many of the foods already recommended in this book, like beans, peas and lentils, nuts and seeds, whole grains, as well as dark green vegetables, like spinach, kale, chard, beet tops, Brussel sprouts and broccoli. Aim for a serving (1 cup raw or 1/2 cup cooked) of these veggies every day and choose plant-based protein foods daily too.

Eating regularly is another key strategy for helping your mood. When we are hungry, we can become irritable (hangry!) and anxious. These are real feelings that I often experience. It's important to tune into your body and these feelings and look at why you may not be eating and if that could be impacting your mood. For me, it ties into my low appetite in the morning and my love of drinking coffee first thing. Although I don't feel hunger, I do notice the sensations in my body and my anxiety creeping in. I have to force myself sometimes, to pause my coffee consumption and eat or drink something, whether a smoothie, *Chia Pudding*, a muffin or just a snack of some fruit and yogurt. Usually, once I take a bite or two, I notice my true hunger and it feels good to eat.

The other time of day I struggle with is in the afternoon, especially if I have not taken the time to have a nourishing lunch. It's usually when I start prepping our family dinner and I think that I can just wait to eat that, but dinner often isn't for another few hours. This is when I will grab a handful of nuts, rather than just open a non-alcoholic beer, and it helps to settle me so I don't become irritable with my family leading up to dinnertime.

Tips for Healing Mood with Food

- Support your neurotransmitters with sufficient protein every meal and snack
- Fill up on omega-3 fats from chia and ground flax seeds, fatty fish or with a supplement
- Focus on folate from legumes, whole grains and green veggies every day

Self-Reflection on your Mood

Recovery is a time of change and it's natural to have ups and downs. Can you find joy in small things, like a pleasurable food, drink or activity? Do you have someone to talk to about how you're feeling or can you write your thoughts down in a journal?

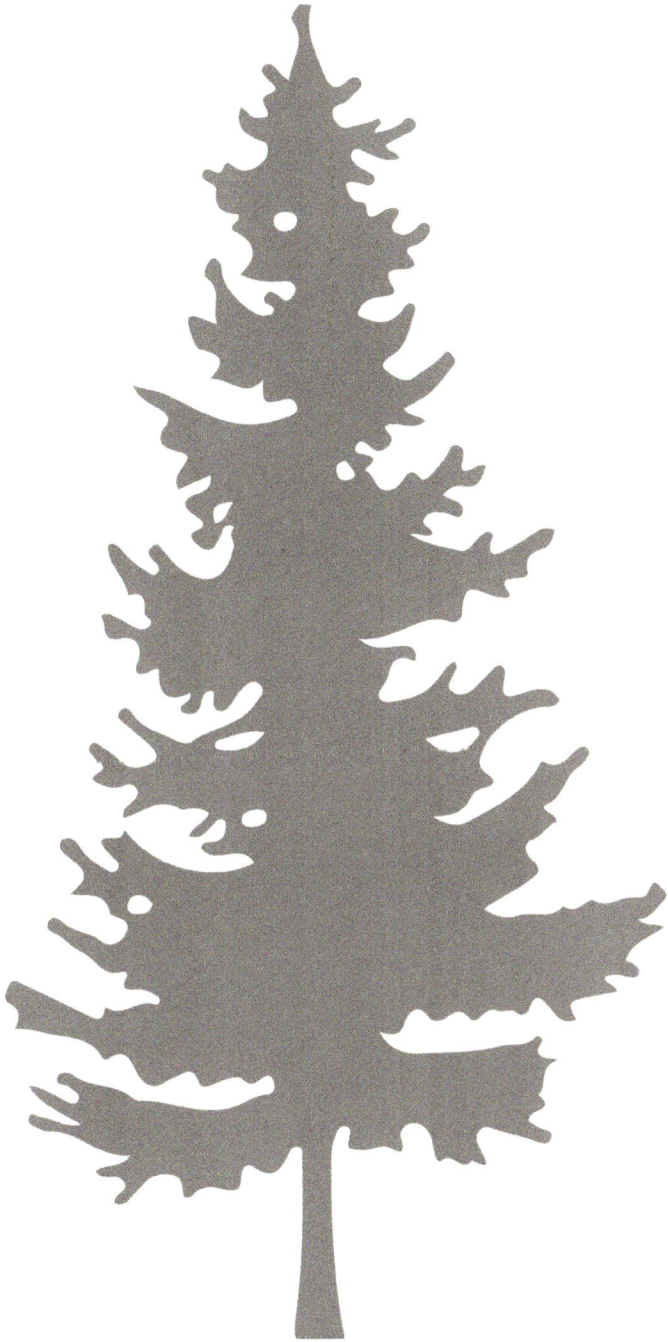

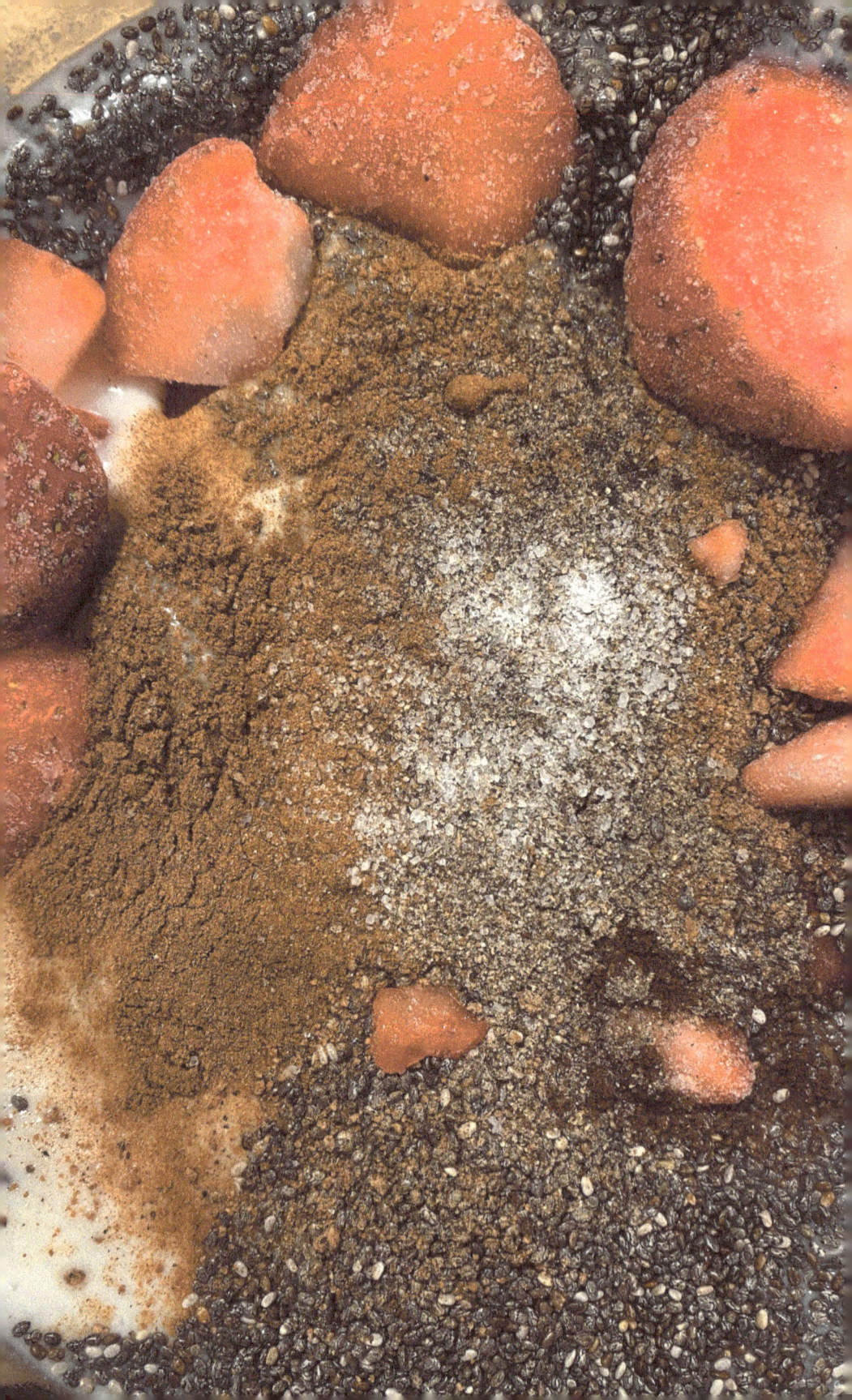

Chia Pudding

To help anyone's gut health and especially provide binding support, chia seeds are packed with soluble fibre and essential omega 3 fats. Keep chia pudding in the refrigerator for up to a week for an easy breakfast or snack.

Serves 4

1/2 cup whole chia seeds   Pinch salt
2 cups milk

Combine all ingredients in an airtight container and let soak in the refrigerator for minimum 2 hours until set. Serve with a drizzle of maple syrup, a sprinkle of cinnamon and your favourite fruit.

Focus On Fluids

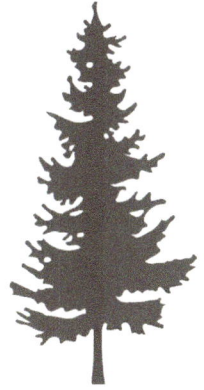

In my treatment for addiction, coffee was the number one fluid consumed by the clients. It was readily available and when giving up other substances, it felt like one thing that could be held onto, especially when feeling the fatigue that comes along with detox.

However, I noticed that when I consumed a few cups of coffee in the morning, it displaced my appetite tor breakfast. And by the time we started our lectures, I was jittery, anxious and restless. None of these feelings are conducive to learning and reflecting, whether about addiction or any other type of learning you might be doing. So I started asking for a carafe of decaf coffee in the mornings and it caught on with many others. It also allowed me to decrease one of my prescribed medications which gave me a sedative-type effect.

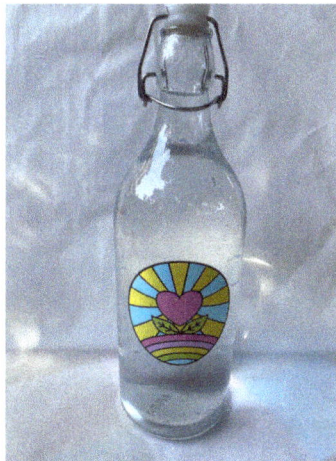

Water is one of the most important nutrients for the body and should be consumed readily throughout detox, recovery and everyday life. The recommendation for adult women is 9 cups and adult men 12 cups per day. Although for many people, plain tap water is not very appealing, which makes the beverage industry billions of dollars. Here are some alternatives to plain tap water that are just as hydrating:

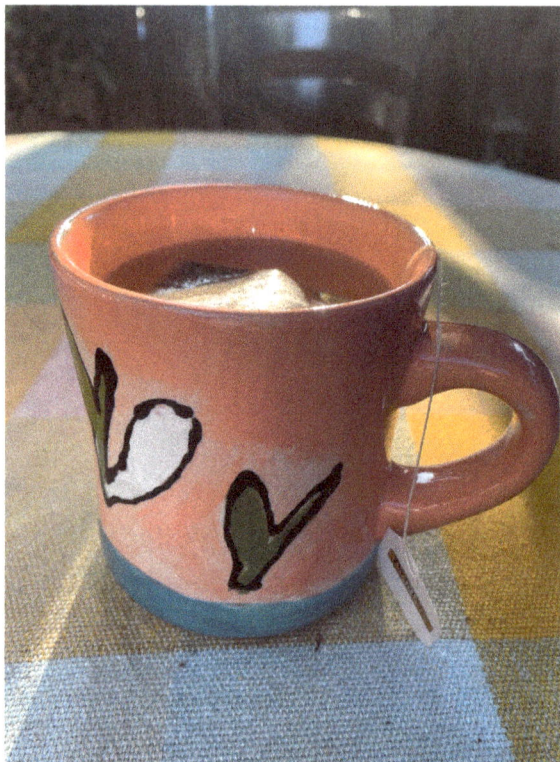

Herbal tea or hot water can help stimulate the movement of the digestive tract. Varieties like ginger or peppermint can be soothing for nausea for some individuals but overall any type of herbal tea that gets you consuming more fluids is a good one. It can also be brewed then chilled for a refreshing cold or iced tea if that is your preference and it is a better choice than store bought iced teas which can contain added sugar and caffeine.

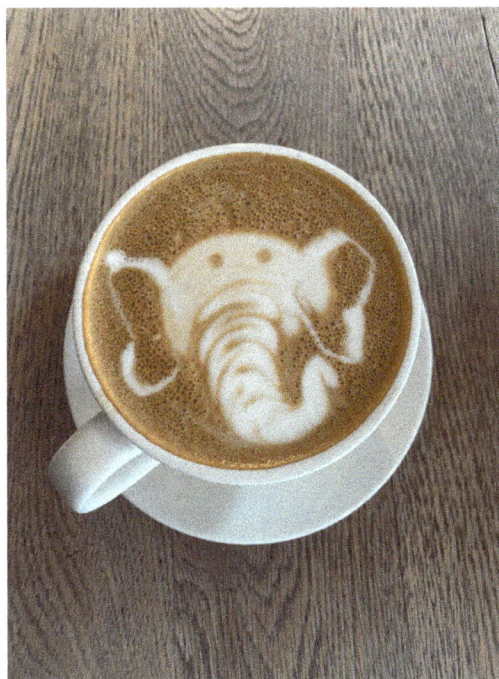

Coffee in moderation can be a hydrating fluid but caffeine in excess can cause anxiety as mentioned, displace appetite and in very high quantities may pose a risk for heart attack. Try decaffeinated coffee or half caf and limit the amount of added sugar and cream, especially flavoured creamers, which can tax the liver.

Juice can be a hydrating fluid but can also contain a lot of natural and sometimes added sugar. Excess fructose (the sugar in fruit) can be hard on the liver and is linked to increased trigylcerides, one of the fats in our body that can impact heart health. Keep juice to no more than 1/2 a cup per day and consider diluting it with water, or making *Nikki-ade* for electrolyte replacement, which you can find at the end of the chapter. Avoid store-bought sports drinks, which are only recommended if you're exercising or sweating for more than an hour.

Many individuals ask about fresh-pressed juices for detoxification, whether in recovery or after the holidays. Vegetable-based juices, like carrot, celery or beet can be a wonderful addition to the diet, especially for those who consume few vegetables or have a low appetite, but eating the vegetables (and fruit) is always better than juicing them, as the fibre is maintained. 1 cup of freshly squeezed orange juice may require up to 10 oranges, but you would never be able to eat that many at once. As well, store-bought vegetable juices contain huge amounts of added sodium as a preservative, so making your own can be a much healthier alternative.

Low blood sugar can occur for those with metabolic disruptions, like diabetes, or for those in withdrawal from substances and low intake of food. Symptoms of low blood sugar can include sweating, anxiety, confusion, shakiness and headache. The fastest way to bring up blood sugar is from a sweetened beverage, like juice, but it's important to eat after consuming it within about 15 minutes or blood sugar will drop rapidly again.

Smoothies, unlike juice, retain all of the fibre from the fruit or vegetables. As fresh veggies and fruit are so hydrating, smoothies can be a great way to get some fluids, fibre and possibly protein depending on what you add like yogurt, kefir, milk or seeds. For a bright *Green Smoothie*, check out the recipe section or use up what you have access too, like berries or bananas, which can also be frozen if they are ripening too quickly.

Milk is a hydrating fluid that also provides protein, calcium and vitamin D. It can be a contentious subject whether adults should consume cow's milk. Some individuals struggle with lactose intolerance, especially as they age. Lactose-free milk is commonly available as a solution. Chocolate milk contains added sugar so should be used in moderation, but it still contains protein, calcium and vitamin D so it is more nutritious than other sugar-sweetened beverages.

Plant-based milk alternatives, like soy, almond, oat, cashew, rice or hemp, can be fortified with calcium, vitamin D and sometimes B12 and they do not contain lactose so some individuals may find them easier to digest. However, the level of protein in these beverages vary dramatically, with only soy being equivalent to cow's milk, followed by oat. Almond, cashew and rice milks have virtually no protein and if using these, other protein sources should be prioritized.

Soda pop is not a recommended fluid in recovery or in life. They contain no nutrients except added sugar, which has been mentioned as a challenge for the liver. The carbonation in these beverages can also be linked to excess gas, belching, reflux and bloating. Use them in moderation as a treat now and again.

Carbonated and mineral waters can be a refreshing alternative to still water and can add extra minerals like calcium and magnesium. Be mindful of the above digestive symptoms, like bloating, if consuming these frequently.

Infused waters can also bring water to life! Add sliced cucumber, fresh herbs, slices of citrus, melon or fresh or frozen berries. If you prepare these in larger quantities, consider investing in a pitcher with a separate steeping container so that you can remove the vegetables or fruit after a few hours before it breaks down too much. This would also be a great addition in a treatment centre to draw clients to consuming more water in place of caffeinated beverages.

Non-alcoholic alternatives are widely available and have become popular with those in recovery as well as other people interested in healthier options. However the decision to consume these is entirely individual. For some people in recovery, these beverages may be too similar to alcoholic versions and can light up dopamine pathways in the brain and become too much of a transition back to consuming the old standards. Many still contain low levels of alcohol (0.5%) which can also be problematic for some in recovery from alcohol, although there are numerous options on the market now that are 0.0% and completely de-alcoholized.

For others they are a safe alternative and provide options for consuming similar beverages at social gatherings and restaurants. One or two non-alcoholic beers, glasses of wine or mocktails can be more fun for some than drinking water and they taste very similar. Many conventional alcohol companies are offering non-alcoholic counterparts. Use them cautiously at first and always ask yourself why you are choosing them and if they are negatively affecting your recovery. With less sugar and calories than alcoholic beverages, they may drive appetite for some or displace food for others.

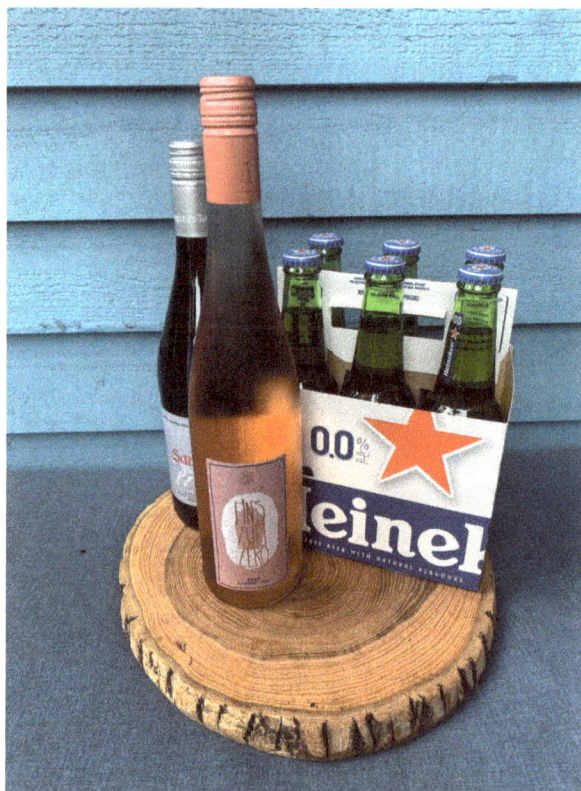

For me, these beverages are one of my key recovery strategies and have allowed me to embrace a life without alcohol. I find they taste exactly the same and give me the same comfort, without messing with my mind. I have found so many non-alcoholic beers, wines, spirits and mocktails and I keep a huge selection in my fridge so it feels like a celebration every time I open it and get to choose one. I've also noticed many of my family members and friends enjoying these beverages, sometimes to support me, and also for their own moderation. For the first time in decades, alcohol consumption is on the decline in Canada.

Tips to Focus on Fluids

- Drink healthy fluids often throughout the day to maintain your hydration
- Be cautious with caffeinated beverages, like coffee and cola, that can increase anxiety and sleep disturbances and displace appetite
- Find alternatives to alcohol that work for you and bring you joy

Self-Reflection on Your Hydration

Up to 60% of the human body is water so give your cells and organs what they need to survive. Can you find a beverage or two that bring you the joy that alcohol did? Do you need a fluid tracker to remind you to drink healthy beverages regularly throughout the day?

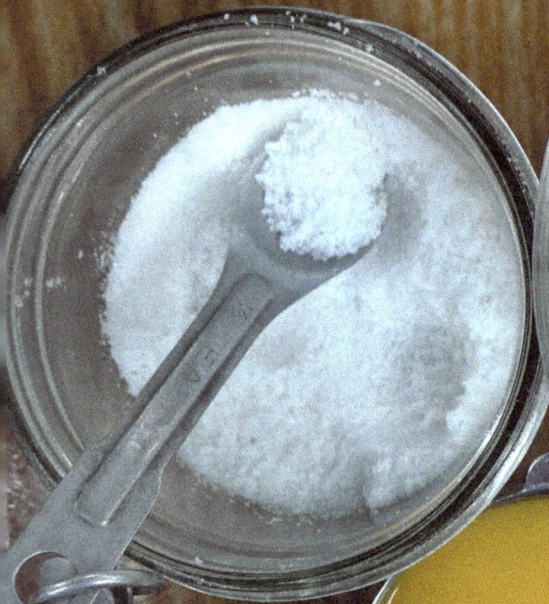

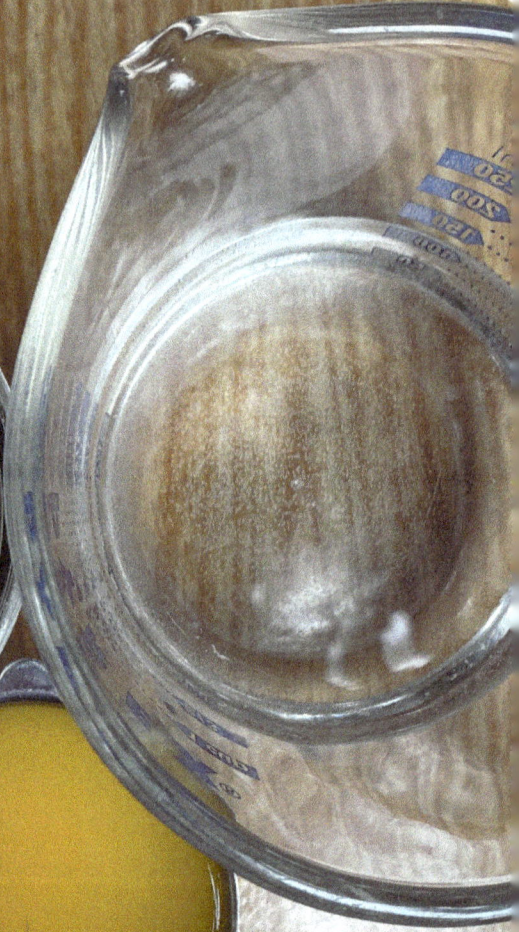

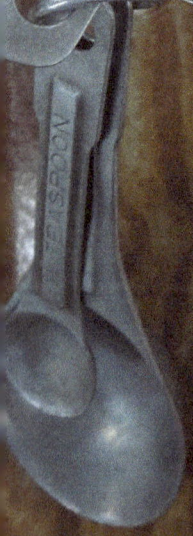

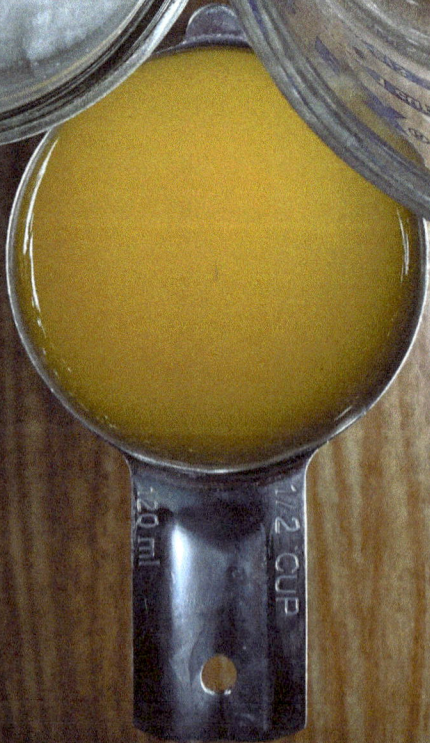

Nikki-Ade Electrolyte Replacement

A much more affordable and natural alternative to store-bought electrolyte replacement beverages, this ratio of juice to water allows for optimum uptake of the fluid and sugar for a quick burst of energy and hydration.

1 serving

1/2 cup juice (orange is good
for potassium)

1/2 cup water
1/2 tsp salt

Combine together and drink liberally.

Dietary Restrictions

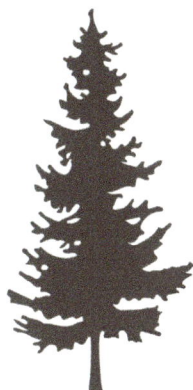

There are a variety of different dietary restrictions that individuals experience, ranging from those essential for health to those required by religion or chosen for ethical or sustainability values. This section may be of use for those preparing food in treatment centres or sober-living houses.

Food allergy is the most severe restriction and it is required by those with anaphylactic, life-threatening allergies to certain foods, often nuts or seafood. It has been shown that up to 7% of the Canadian population suffers from these severe food allergies and they are often diagnosed early in life and require strict avoidance of the food, including cross-contamination, where trace amounts are unintentionally added to a food that should not contain the allergen. Reactions can range from itching in the mouth or skin (e.g hives) to nausea, vomiting, diarrhea to swelling of the air passage and changes to the circulatory system.

Those with anaphylactic allergy should carry epinephrine auto-injectors at all times because if they do ingest their food allergen, life-threatening reactions, like the airway closing or blood pressure dropping, can happen within minutes. And each reaction may be worse than the last as the immune system wages a stronger response. Epinephrine (adrenaline) is the only recommended treatment in cases of anaphylaxis, not anti-histamines. Treatment centres and sober-living houses should have stock epinephrine available as best practice, in case a client forgets their own or require a higher dose.

Food intolerance is suffered by a much higher percentage of individuals, and it is not life-threatening, but can be extremely uncomfortable. Digestive upset can be the most common symptom, but others may experience skin issues, head or muscle aches, fatigue or brain fog. Determining the cause of food intolerance can be very challenging. It often requires a strict elimination diet where very simple and few foods are consumed until symptoms resolve and then foods are challenged one at a time to allow the individual to assess which might be triggering their symptoms.

Some of the common food intolerances include lactose (the natural sugar in milk), which can trigger bloating, pain, gas and diarrhea. Wheat may be another food that individuals may not tolerate well, causing bloating, diarrhea or constipation, brain fog, fatigue or skin issues.

Food intolerance is usually volumetric, meaning individuals can often tolerate small quantities of the food, unlike in allergy, where even trace particles can trigger reactions. Some individuals can also tolerate variations on the food, like dairy if it is fermented (e.g. yogurt not fluid milk) or sourdough (fermented) bread, rather than yeast-risen bread. Some of those with wheat intolerance can also better manage ancient wheat varietals like spelt, kamut or red fife.

One treatment for those with many food intolerances related to a condition called Irritable Bowel Syndrome (IBS), is the low FODMAP diet. This diet excludes many different foods that contain fermentable sugars and starches, of which lactose sugar and the starch in wheat are included. But there are many other foods that can bother those with IBS, including onion, garlic, certain fruits and vegetables, legumes and even large amounts of nuts. It is recommended to work with a Registered Dietitian to manage IBS and help uncover which foods trigger reactions and what strategies can be used to help heal the irritation in the gut.

Oral allergy syndrome is a condition where individuals react to the protein in the skin of certain raw fruit and vegetables, especially apples, peaches, plums and pears. The mouth and throat become very itchy and irritated. By peeling and cooking the fruit, the protein becomes altered and the reaction does not happen. Some individuals do outgrow this allergy and may be able to consume raw fruit again as they get older.

Celiac disease and gluten intolerance affects many people in North America. Celiac disease is an auto-immune condition where the body attacks itself when gluten is present in the intestine or on the skin. The only management of celiac disease is strict gluten avoidance, including cross-contamination and trace amounts. Gluten is found in wheat (including ancient varietals like spelt, kamut and red fife), barley and rye, as well as their derivatives. It can also be found in hidden ingredients in processed foods and body care products. Those with celiac disease should work with a Gastroenterologist and a Registered Dietitian for blood testing, digestive assessment and dietary management.

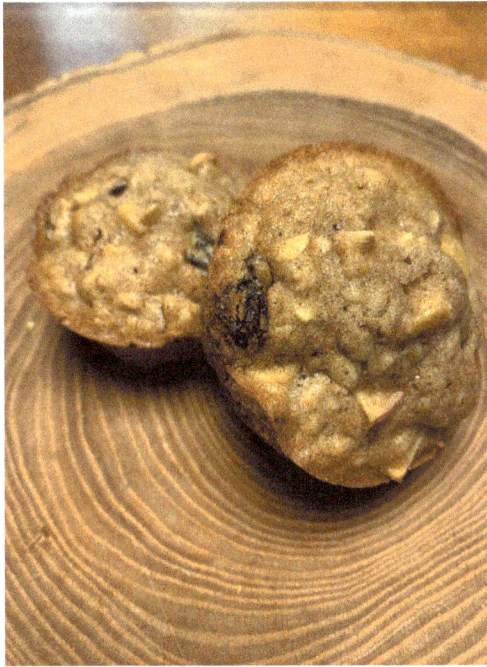

Gluten intolerance is more common than celiac disease but is not as threatening to issues like fertility and cancer risk. It can be very uncomfortable with digestive upset, skin issues, brain fog and fatigue. Cross-contamination is less of an issue and there are many gluten-free products on the market that make eating less gluten easy. Choose gluten-free 1:1 flour for easy substitutions in baking, find your favourite gluten-free bread, crackers and noodles. And opt for naturally gluten-free grains and grain products made from rice, corn, quinoa, millet and gluten-free oats.

I have gained a much closer understanding of gluten-free diets since my daughter was tested for celiac disease and showed an elevated blood marker. She underwent two endoscopies to assess the health of her digestive tract, but those tests came back negative. My guess is that we just discovered this sensitivity to gluten very early due to my knowledge and advocacy for testing as a dietitian. Although the surgeon said she could keep eating gluten, it didn't feel right to me to keep feeding it to her when she was reacting to it and not absorbing iron and vitamin D sufficiently to meet her needs.

So we went gluten-free at home, although she continues to be a "normal" kid when she's out with friends, which is very important for her at this age. We only buy gluten-free bread, crackers and noodles and we have found some amazing alternatives. Our weekly menu has changed from a lot of pasta to more rice and quinoa bowls, corn tortillas for taco night instead of burrito shells. And the best news is that it is working and her blood marker for celiac disease has almost normalized!

Other health considerations may be due to chronic diseases or the risk of them. Some may choose a predominantly plant-based diet because of issues like high cholesterol. Those with diabetes need to manage their intake of starch and grain foods as well as sugar. It is recommended to work with a Registered Dietitian to meal plan for these types of restrictions. Check the final chapter on **Resources** for support.

Religious restrictions, like eating Halal as in the Muslim religion or eating Kosher as in the Jewish religion, require avoidance of certain foods like pork. They also require that animal foods be blessed during the slaughtering process, so the meats that are allowable, such as poultry and beef, must be certified Halal or Kosher. Some strict Muslims or Jews require foods to be prepared in a certain manner, with certain food combinations not allowed and prevention of contamination by non-Halal or non-Kosher ingredients (e.g. needing a separate kitchen).

Ethical considerations may be the reason some individuals choose vegan or plant-based diets, as an objection to the killing or keeping of animals for human use. Strict vegans avoid all animal foods, including dairy products, as well as honey. Some hidden ingredients to be aware of include gelatine, which is made from pork or beef bones and lecithin, which may be made from eggs but can be made from soy (check the package). Whey and casein are the proteins in milk and may be found in high protein processed foods, like bars or powders.

Sustainability restrictions may be the reason some people choose certain foods, as our food choices are one of the number one causes of climate change. They might opt for sustainably raised or harvested animal foods or organically grown fruits and vegetables. This can be a challenge for those living in treatment centres due to the (often) higher cost of foods which can be out of the budget limitations. Sustainability is a very important topic so please see the chapter on **Sustainability** to understand more.

With any dietary restriction, it is an individualized approach in home cooking or those in treatment centres, with some requiring much more strict management. The requirements are much different for those in commercial food preparation.

Tips for Dietary Restrictions

- Seek support for managing your symptoms or dietary restrictions from healthcare professionals or food providers
- Understand whether you need to limit or completely avoid certain foods
- For food providers, work closely with your clients, to meet their needs in an inclusive and nutritious way

Self-Reflection on Your Dietary Considerations

Your food choices are your own so take responsibility and advocate for what your body needs. Do you need to ask for support to get the nutrition that works for you?

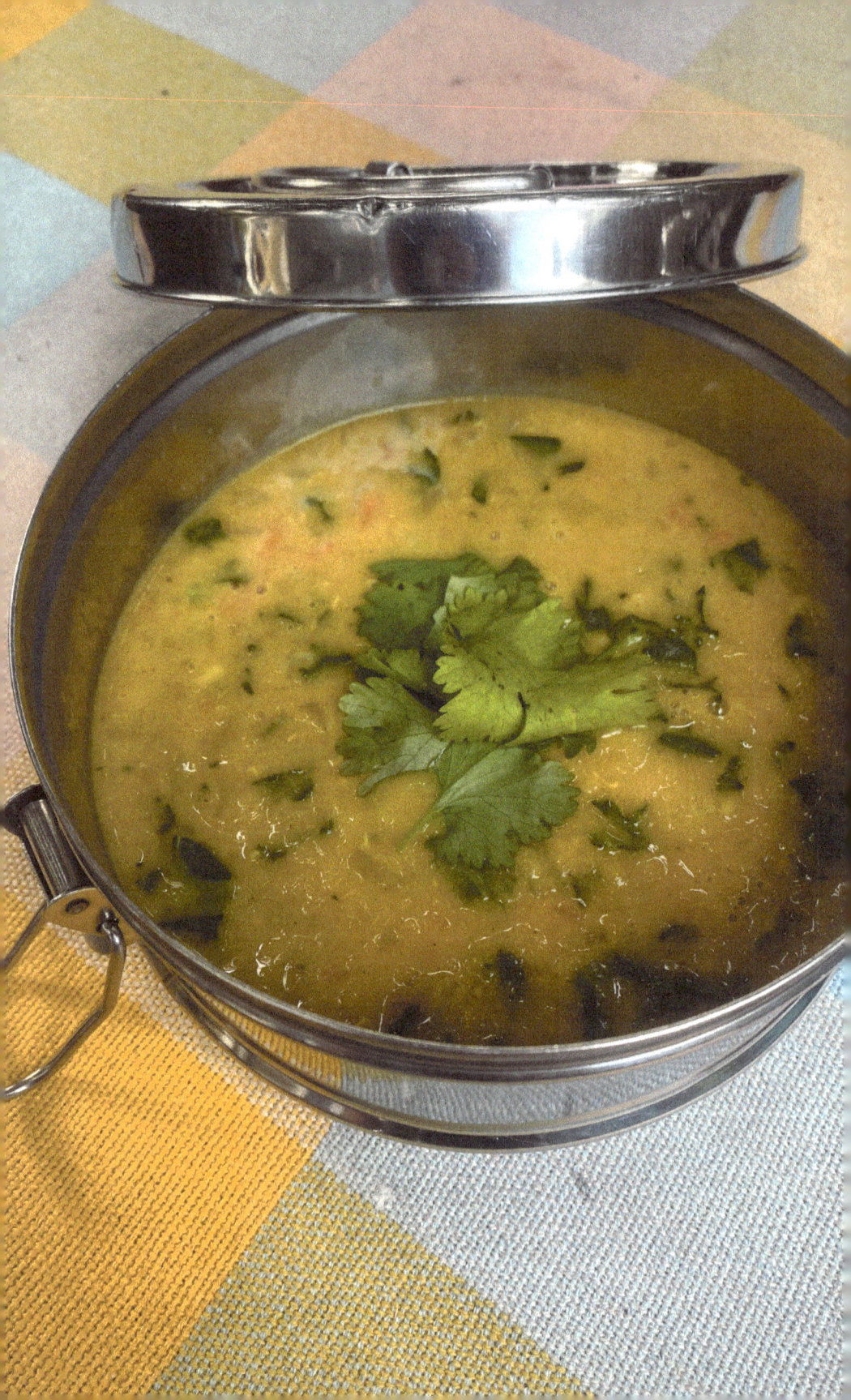

Lentil Soup

A comforting meal filled with fibre and plant-based protein. Learning the basics of soup-making can provide the skills needed to make a nourishing meal out of any vegetables you may be able to access. For those needing an even simpler meal, use a starter canned or packaged version, but soup it up by adding canned legumes and extra veggies.

Serves 4

2 Tbsp olive oil
1 onion, finely chopped
2 stalks celery, finely chopped
1 large carrot, finely chopped
3 cloves garlic, minced or pressed
1 cup red lentils
1 tsp salt

6 cups water or vegetable stock
1 bay leaf
Additional veggies as desired
(e.g. 2 cups chopped spinach or
kale, 1 large chopped potato or
sweet potato)

Heat a large pot on medium low heat, then add the oil. Saute onion, celery, carrot and garlic until softened and golden. Add lentils, salt, water or stock and bay leaf. Bring to a boil then reduce heat and simmer until lentils are soft, approximately 30 minutes. Add additional veggies if using and cook until soft. Serve hot with a side of whole grain bread. Refrigerate leftovers for up to 5 days or freeze for up to 3 months.

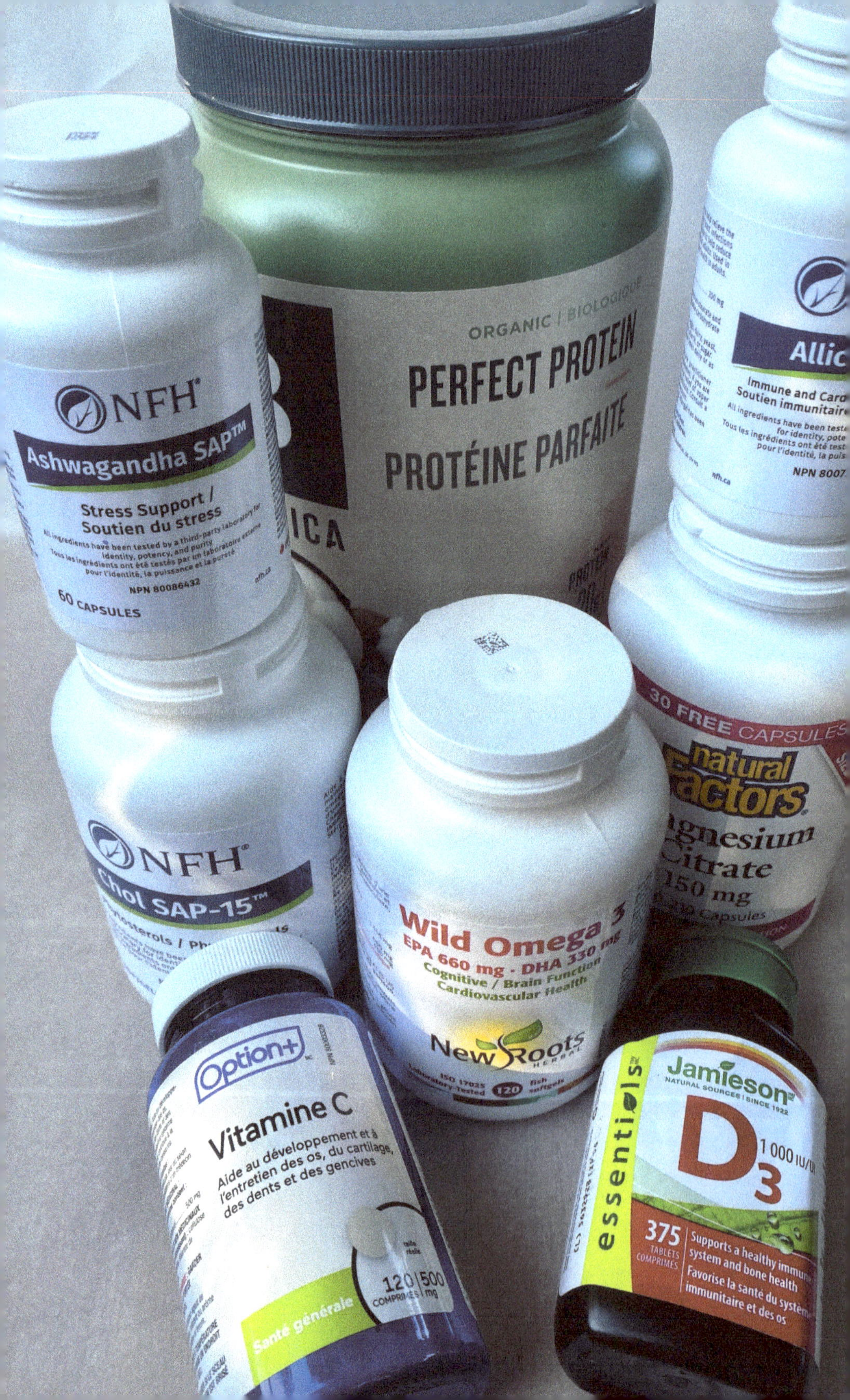
ORGANIC | BIOLOGIQUE
PERFECT PROTEIN
PROTÉINE PARFAITE
NFH
Ashwagandha SAP™
Stress Support /
Soutien du stress
60 CAPSULES
NPN 80086432
Immune and Card
Soutien immunitaire
NPN 8007
NFH
Chol SAP-15™
30 FREE CAPSULES
natural factors
Magnesium Citrate
150 mg
Wild Omega 3
EPA 660 mg · DHA 330 mg
Cognitive / Brain Function
Cardiovascular Health
New Roots
120
Option+
Vitamine C
Aide au développement et à l'entretien des os, du cartilage, des dents et des gencives
120 | 500 mg
Santé générale
Jamieson
D3
1 000 IU
essentials
375
Supports a healthy immune system and bone health
Favorise la santé du système immunitaire et des os

Supplementation

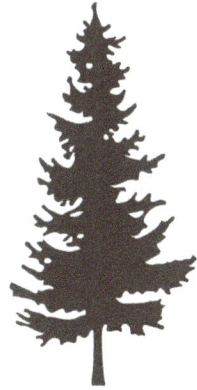

In substance abuse, we often deplete our bodies of essential nutrients by displacing food with alcohol, suppressing appetite with stimulants or being so dysfunctional that we cannot cook for ourselves or prioritize nourishing our bodies.

So in recovery, it is key to build back the body's stores and consume optimal levels of nutrients to restore functioning and allow the body and mind to thrive. As mentioned in the first chapter on **Detoxification**, there are some nutrients that are standard practice in the first days of withdrawal. These are usually supplemented to ensure adequate intake, when eating food can be a challenge due to nausea, vomiting, fatigue and other symptoms. Supplement amounts have been determined by Canada's Recommended Dietary Allowances (see **References**).

Thiamine, or vitamin B1, is required by the body to metabolize carbohydrates and for proper nerve function. It can be found readily in whole grains, legumes, nuts and meat, although supplementation is recommended for alcohol withdrawal in the range of 250-500 mg/day. To support continued B1 needs, consider soft, easily digestible foods like oatmeal, brown rice congee, lentil soup or peanut butter on whole grain bread.

Vitamin B12 is required for cells to function properly and for DNA formation as well as for nervous system functions in the body. It is harder to find in plant-based food choices, with the only sources being nutritional yeast, which is a flavourful ingredient that can be used as a popcorn topping in place of salt as well as added for a punch of umami flavour to sauces, soups, stews and in breading. Fortified vegan foods, like plant-based milk alternatives and vegan meat alternatives, like veggie dogs, may contain B12 and this form of the vitamin can be more absorbable than the B12 that is naturally contained in animal foods.

For those that consume animal foods regularly, B12 is usually not a concern. But as we age and for those with stomach conditions, we may not produce enough of the stomach acid necessary to cleave B12 from protein which means it cannot be absorbed by the body.

Those who do not consume animal foods, as well as older adults or those with stomach problems should take a regular B12 supplement of 2.4 micrograms per day.

Vitamin C is a key component of the immune system and an antioxidant, helping fight free radicals in our body that are linked to cardiovascular disease and cancer. Vitamin C is abundant in fresh fruits and vegetables and if we consume this as half of our plate at most meals and snacks, we take in a sufficient amount. Vitamin C is degraded by heat and lost in water so when we cook these fruits and vegetables, we do not get as much vitamin C.

Vitamin C supplements, whether tablets or powdered, are commonly consumed as it may be tempting to assume we need these to boost our immune health. Research shows however that vitamin C does not prevent the common cold, except in rare circumstances like extremely cold climates.

Instead, excess vitamin C in supplement form can have unpleasant side effects like digestive upset and diarrhea. As well, vitamin C is a water-soluble vitamin that is not stored in body so when we consume more than our body can use, our body excretes it in urine. Fresh fruits and vegetables can easily provide enough vitamin C so it is a better choice to consume these daily to get what we need.

Cigarette smokers require more vitamin C than non-smokers due to the higher amount of free radicals produced in the body from smoking. If not consuming fresh fruits and vegetables at most meals, consider a supplement of no more than 1,000 milligrams per day.

Vitamin D plays many roles in the body, helping us build bone, hormones and in the immune system. Vitamin D is very low in the food supply, with only fatty fish and egg yolks being sources of it. In Canada, cow's milk, as well as many other plant-based milk alternatives, are fortified with this vitamin. However, it is still recommended for most Canadians to supplement with vitamin D, at 1,000 IU per day for adults (and 2,000 IU per day for older adults), especially during the months of October to April when the sun is not strong enough for us to produce it in our skin.

Vitamin D is known as the "sunshine" vitamin because when UV rays from the sun are strong enough, we produce an abundance in our skin. That said, when we wear sunscreen, which is important for protecting against skin cancer, or for those with darker skin pigments, we do not produce vitamin D and so supplementation is key.

Iron is a mineral required in our body for the production of red blood cells. This means it is essential for us to get the oxygen our cells need and for us to feel energetic. Fatigue and pallor are common symptom of iron deficiency, but it can also be expressed as anxiety for some. Iron is the most common nutrient deficiency around the world, especially for women and children.

Iron is found in most protein foods, except for dairy. The iron in animal proteins is more readily absorbed by the body but iron is plentiful in plant protein foods as well. The iron in plants is more absorbable by the body when it is consumed along with vitamin C. Try adding fresh fruits and vegetables, for vitamin C, along with plant-based protein foods for iron. For example, add red pepper or orange segments to spinach salad or tomatoes along with beans, peas and lentils or snack on apple and peanut butter.

For those that do not consume animal foods or for those with diagnosed iron deficiency, it is recommended to take a supplement of 50-150mg of elemental iron. New research shows that when we take high levels of iron supplements daily, our bodies down regulate absorption because it thinks iron is plentiful. The recommendation is take iron supplements every other day. Iron supplements can also cause digestive upset and constipation so by taking it every other day and ensuring adequate fluid and fibre in the amount of 30-35 g per day, we can help manage these side effects.

Calcium is the mineral that forms our bones and inadequate intake quickly causes the body to break down bone faster to keep blood calcium levels stable. The richest source of calcium is in dairy foods, like milk, yogurt and cheese. Calcium is also found in plant foods like sesame, almond, navy beans, tofu and dark green vegetables, like leafy greens and broccoli. Plant-based milk alternatives are usually fortified with calcium to make the levels equivalent to cow's milk.

Calcium needs do increase as we age, after menopause for women and after age 70 for men. It can be difficult to meet these needs from food alone, so a supplement may be warranted. It is recommended to take lower levels of calcium supplements more than once per day, for example 250-500 mg with two separate meals. Avoid taking 1,000 mg of calcium as a supplement at one time.

Magnesium is also a key component of bone health as well as performing hundreds of other functions in the body. Magnesium is abundant in the food supply, if we cook mostly at home and consume minimally processed foods. Rich sources include nuts, seeds, beans, peas, lentils, whole grains and dark green leafy vegetables. Include these foods daily or consider a supplement, especially as a remedy for muscle spasms, headache or constipation. Many bone health supplements package magnesium along with calcium, but be cautious with high doses of magnesium in supplement form as they can cause digestive upset and diarrhea. 150 mg of magnesium per day in the form of magnesium citrate is an amount tolerated by most people. We cannot take in too much magnesium from food sources however.

Omega 3 is an essential fat that our body cannot make and it can be hard to get from the food supply. It is known to reduce inflammation in our bodies, as well as be key for brain, heart, skin and immune health. The only sources are fatty fish, like salmon, trout, sardines and herring as well as ground flax, chia seeds and hemp hearts. Choose fatty fish at least twice per week or consume 2 Tbsp of these seeds daily, which have the added benefit of soluble fibre for gut and heart health. If these foods are not regularly consumed, an omega 3 supplement is another option. There are omega 3 supplements derived from fish (e.g. fish oil) or from plant sources like algae in the range of 1000 mg per day. Try to choose sustainable versions that do not deplete our fish supply and degrade our waterways.

Protein is a nutrient that is abundant in most of our diets, despite what the food industry and the many "high-protein" processed foods may lead you to believe. Protein is an essential building block for muscle, organs, as well as all of our body's chemical messengers and compounds like neurotransmitters in the brain, hormones and enzymes. Aim to consume protein at all meals and snacks as approximately 1/4 of your plate and choose protein from plant sources most often. Excess animal protein, especially from red, grilled and preserved meats, is linked to cardiovascular disease and certain cancers, especially colon cancer.

You can take in too much protein and this can be hard on the liver and kidneys that have to process it, if excess consumption is long term. Protein breakdown produces ammonia, which is a toxin in the body and has to be converted to urea and excreted by the kidneys in our urine. As mentioned excess animal protein is also linked to cardiovascular disease and certain cancers. It is rare to consume excess protein from plant sources. The average amount needed by adults is 1 gram per kilogram of body weight with amounts of 1.5 grams/kg recommended for those needing to build muscle, fight infection and heal wounds. 2 grams/kg is the highest level recommended and should not be consumed long term.

Despite what the fitness industry portrays, it is harder to build muscle in a calorie deficit (cutting) so be sure you are also consuming healthy carbohydrates (e.g. whole grains, fruits and vegetables) and healthy fats from plants or fish along with your protein. After a workout, to optimize muscle, consume a protein-rich meal within one hour. If carbohydrates are not consumed along with the protein, the body will break the protein down as energy, to replace the fuel stores in our muscles and liver that have been used in exercise.

Multivitamin and mineral supplements are very commonly consumed and may seem like an insurance policy against a poor diet. However, many of the nutrients in multivitamins are not needed if you are consuming a balanced diet and they are not stored in the body, so you excrete them in your urine. Rather than take a multivitamin, follow the food recommendations in this book and work with a health professional, like a Registered Dietitian, to determine if specific vitamin or mineral supplements may be beneficial for you depending on your age, health condition or wellness goals.

Other supplements, like herbal remedies, are plentiful and targeted towards a myriad of symptoms, health conditions and stages of life. Be cautious with over consuming supplements or looking for a "miracle" pill. Work closely with your healthcare professional to determine which supplements may be right for you to manage your health concerns and to avoid interfering with medications you may be taking.

In treatment centres, it is common to be supplemented with B vitamins, as they are commonly low in alcoholics. But to get other supplements requires advocacy on the part of the client and this was much easier for me as a dietitian, who had lab values to back up my requests. As a predominantly plant-based eater, my vitamin B12 value has been a concern, so I take it regularly. I also take vitamin D, which is recommended for all Canadians, and more so for those struggling with addiction who may be isolating at home and not getting sun exposure, even in the summer months.

I also struggle with high LDL ("lousy") cholesterol, which is ironic as a plant-forward eater who consumes very little saturated fat (which is linked to high LDL cholesterol) and being a dietitian, but clearly has genetic foundations for me. To combat this, I take omega 3 and plant sterol supplements, but please work with your healthcare provider to determine which supplements are right for you and your health goals.

Tips for Supplementation

- Food is always preferred over supplements
- Consider the nutrients that may be lacking in your diet or needed by your body in higher ways than the food you are eating can provide and supplement those specifically
- Take your supplements at ideal times to benefit their absorption, some with food and some spaced at different times in the day

Self-Reflection on Supplements

Supplements cannot replace the need for nutritious food. Do you eat a balanced diet with half your plate fruits and veggies? Do you have any health or food conditions that may require more nutrients than food can provide?

Activity And Exercise

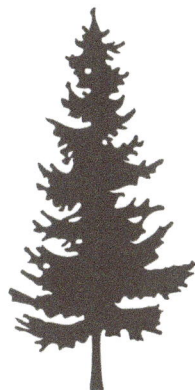

This book is focused on nourishing your body with good food but one of the other key facets of optimal physical and mental health is getting enough exercise. Physical activity is linked to improved health in so many ways, from cardiovascular to bone to brain. The research shows that physical activity can relieve symptoms of depression and anxiety in better ways for some than medications and the best part is there can be very few side effects or costs associated with being active.

The Canadian 24 Hour Movement Guidelines recommend that adults get 150 minutes of moderate-vigorous exercise per week (in other words, 30 minutes, 5 days a week). They also recommend minimizing sedentary time by doing light activity like walking and reducing the time sitting down. Take breaks from sitting every 30-60 minutes by stretching, tidying up around the house, talking on the phone or going for a walk.

Moderate to vigorous activity is important for your cardiovascular health and means getting your heart rate up, perhaps a bit of "huffing and puffing". It does not have to be jogging or running on a treadmill, unless that appeals to you. Other suggestions could be playing tennis or basketball, which can be free in many communities at outdoor courts. It could be dancing, whether at home in your living room, or by joining a class. Zumba is a fun, low-pressure type of dance class with different music and simple steps that attracts people from all walks of life.

Cycling can also be a great moderate to vigorous activity and for some, activity that has a purpose, like transportation, can inspire them. Swimming is another choice and has the added benefit of being very easy on the body, especially for those with injury or disease like arthritis. Being submerged in water is also very therapeutic for many. If you enjoy being in water but not the repetitive nature of swimming laps, consider a water aerobics class.

Resistance and strength-building activity is important for maintaining our bone density and preventing osteoporosis as we age. It also helps us build or maintain our muscle mass which keeps our metabolic rate from dropping as we age and helps us prevent falls, which are the key cause of decreased quality of life in older adults. Maintaining muscle and protecting bone are especially important for women, who have less muscle mass than men and experience menopause, when they lose the bone-protecting effect of the hormone estrogen.

Try Barre-style or Pilates classes or workouts, which do low weight, high repetition movements and use your own body weight to build strength. Jumping rope can be great not only as a resistance activity but also for getting our heart rate elevated quickly. For some lifting weights, at home or at the gym, can be enjoyable.

Barre classes are my favourite activity and I have built it into my recovery, going to one every other day. I love the community at my studio and I am motivated by the strength and tone I have gained, which is key for a peri-menopausal woman. I also love to dance and have a goal of boosting my cardiovascular fitness by attending dance classes or at least putting on some favourite music for an impromptu kitchen dance party.

Outdoor activity is even more linked to improved mood so consider getting out in nature for a walk in a park, the forest or at the beach. Some people like to be active alone but there are many benefits to doing it with others. For one, accountability! It can be easier to stay home and cozy up, especially if the weather is lousy, unless you have someone you have planned to meet up with.

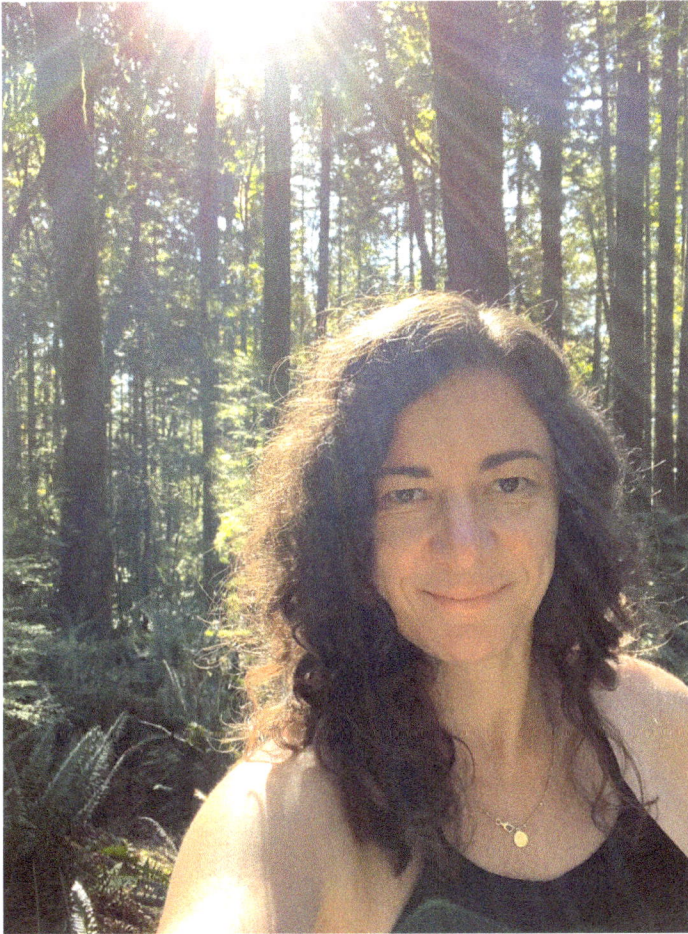

Walking in nature is something I love but don't prioritize nearly enough. It was a wonderful part of the treatment centre I attended which was surrounded by beautiful forests. It's the perfect place for me to pray to the trees, feel the warm sun on my face and hear the birds chirping or the rushing of a stream.

Stretching and balance activity is important for keeping us flexible and preventing injury from sport, exercise or even activities of daily living. Yoga is one of the most well-known stretching activities and has been a cultural practice in India for centuries. There are many styles of yoga from restorative, Yin or Hatha which are slower paced to Flow or hot yoga which can elevate the heart rate. Try different classes or watch online videos from your own home to find the style you enjoy or mix it up. Yoga is also great to improve balance, which will also help us in preventing falls as we age. It can also be incredibly meditative, allowing us to connect to our breath and our bodies and clear our minds.

I love hot yoga, especially in the colder months. For me, it combines stretching with a workout and meditation. And all that sweating feels like it is ridding my body of toxins. But I also enjoyed the yoga classes they offered at the treatment centre and the incredible instructor who held so much wisdom about the practice. It was a very calming time in a period of extreme change and it helped to connect me to my body, which is key in recovery.

Eating before and after exercise is key to optimize energy levels and muscle maintenance. Before exercising, consume easily digestible carbohydrates to give you energy without leaving you feeling too full. A smoothie, yogurt and fruit or a homemade muffin are good suggestions.

After exercising, it is key to consume good carbohydrates, like those from antioxidant-rich fruits and vegetables to help with recovery, along with protein for muscle maintenance. Rather than just having a protein shake, aim for a balanced meal, or if choosing a supplement, opt for a meal replacement beverage that contains carbohydrates, healthy fats as well as protein. If we don't consume carbohydrates after exercising, we will use the protein we consume as energy to replace the glycogen (energy) stores we used up from our muscles and liver, instead of using the protein to repair our muscles.

Tips for Your Activity

- Move your body every day in ways that give you pleasure, whether walking in nature, dancing in the kitchen or going to the gym
- Get up and move around or stretch at least once per hour
- Fuel your body with the nutrients it needs to support activity

Self-Reflection on Your Activity

Our bodies were made to move. Are there reasons why you limit your activity? Can you find one activity this week that would bring you joy and that could be added in regularly?

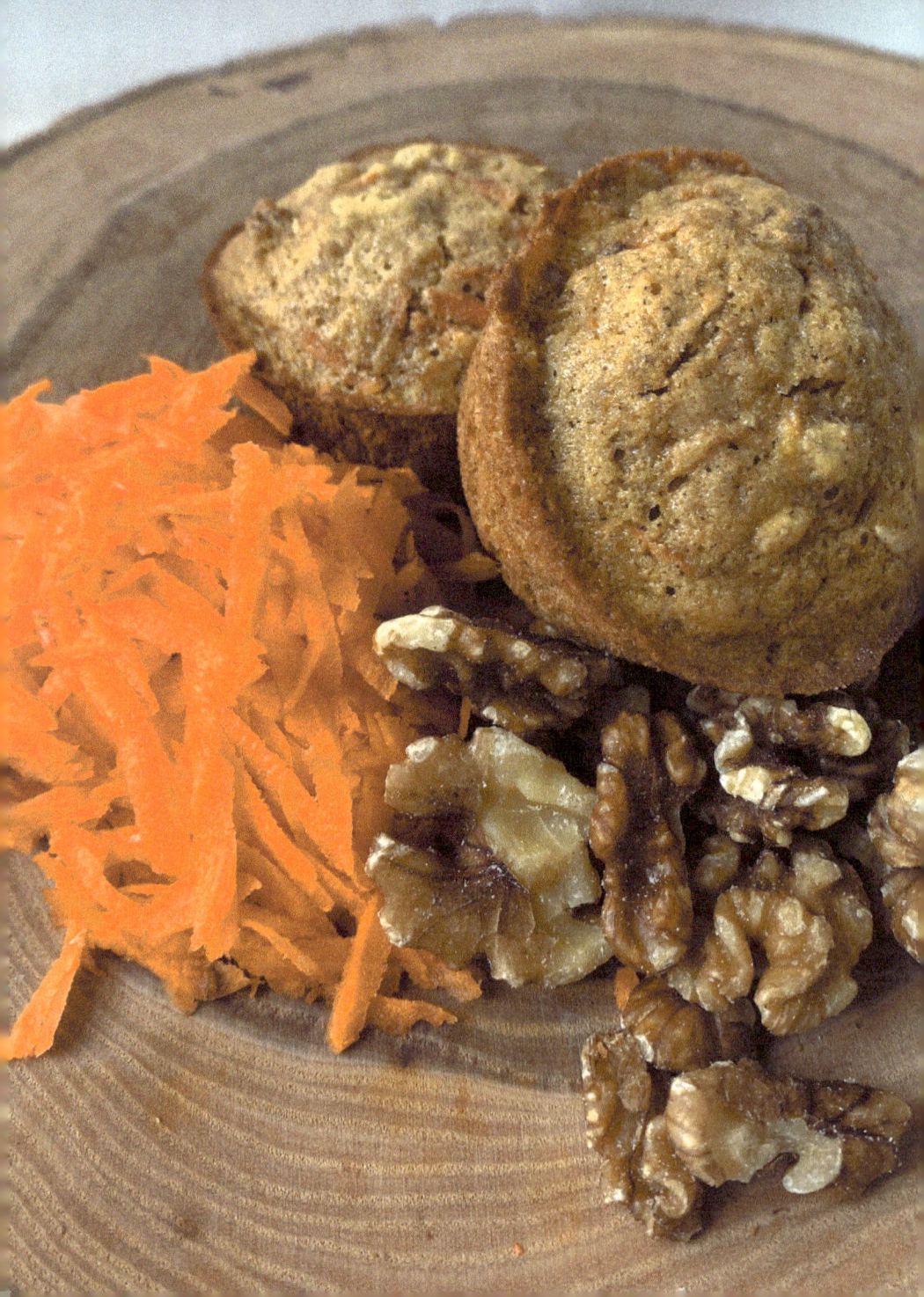

Carrot Muffins

Muffins are so adaptable to the fruit, vegetables and nuts you need to use up. Freeze them for an easy breakfast or snack filled with fibre.

Makes 12 muffins

1/2 cup olive oil
1/2 cup sugar
1 egg
1/2 cup + 2 Tbsps milk
1/2 tsp vanilla
2 cups fruit, vegetables and/or chopped nuts (e.g. grated carrot, canned pumpkin, fresh or frozen berries, peeled/chopped apple or pear; walnuts, pecans)
2 cups flour (whole grain, ground oats or a 1:1 gluten-free mix)
1 tsp baking powder
1/4 tsp baking soda
1/4 tsp salt
1/2 tsp cinnamon
1/2 cup raisins (optional)

Preheat oven to 350F and grease or line a 12 cup muffin tin. In a large bowl, whisk together the oil, sugar, egg, milk and vanilla. Stir in the fruit, vegetables and/or nuts. In a small bowl, combine dry ingredients then add to the wet ingredients, stirring just to combine. Divide into the 12 muffin cups. Bake for 25 minutes until a toothpick inserted comes out clean. Remove to a rack to cool. Store in an air-tight container for up to 3 days or freeze in a tightly sealed bag for up to 3 months.

Sustainability

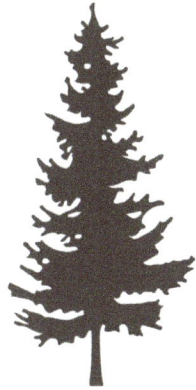

Our food system is one of the leading causes of climate change, but it is often overlooked compared to other issues like transportation and fossil fuels. However, the food choices we make, especially consuming plant-based diets, can have a much greater impact than other common sustainability practices like recycling or LED light bulbs. I dedicate an entire chapter to this integral topic because it is how I choose to eat and I believe in raising awareness about these issues.

Eating sustainably can be a way to be mindful about our food choices and connect us more to our wellbeing goals, both physical and mental, that is a key component of successful recovery. It is also a way to think beyond ourselves, to the wider world and this amazing planet that I hope will thrive for generations to come. This ties into the AA tenet of finding faith in something greater than ourselves and if God is not for you, like it isn't for me, then nature might be your "church" and something to believe in.

Sustainable seafood is raised or harvested in manners that protect our rivers, lakes and oceans. Some fishing methods, like bottom-trawling, cause degradation of the ocean floor, which kills off the vital plants that sea life needs to survive. By-catch is another concern, where unintended species are caught and lost in the process of fishing for edible species. Farmed fish can be another issue with ocean or lake-based farms contaminating the water and wreaking havoc on wild species. But not all farmed seafood is detrimental. Land-based aquaculture can be done in a sustainable manner, where fish are not overcrowded, additives like antibiotics can be lessened and by products are not released into areas that effect wild species.

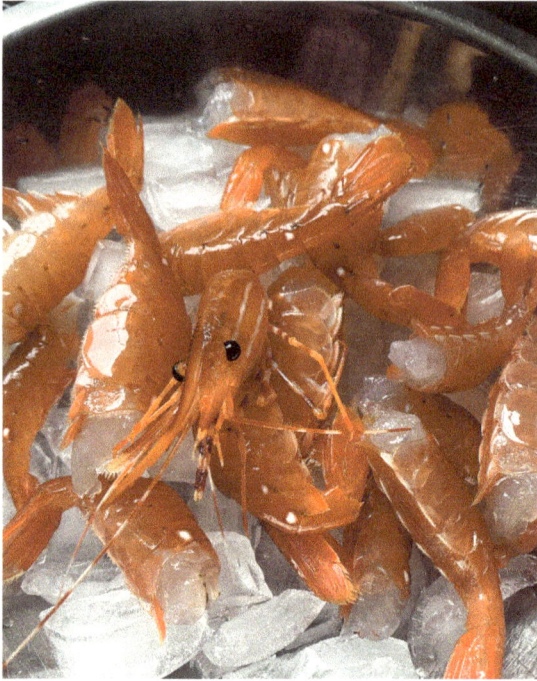

Sustainable meats, poultry, eggs and dairy include grass-fed or wild meats, like bison or venison. These animals graze on their natural diet of grasses, rather than in factory farms where they are fed vast amounts of inexpensive commodity crops like soy and corn. These crops fatten the animals up quickly to increase production and make companies and farmers more money, however ruminant animals like cows are not designed to eat grains. When they rely on these foods instead of grasses, they can develop digestive conditions like metabolic acidosis which then requires antibiotics for treatment.

When choosing red meat and dairy, opt for grass fed or wild meats as often as possible. If those are not available, try to know the source of the meat, like purchasing from a local farm. Organic animal foods also have much stricter standards, with animal welfare being a key concern and certain additives, like growth hormones banned.

With conventional poultry raising, chickens are kept in horrifying conditions, crammed into cages or overcrowded in giant barns. They can be genetically malformed with massive breasts that their legs cannot support or have extensive tumour development. When choosing eggs and poultry, opt for free-range, meaning the birds have at least some access to the outdoors. Again, try to know the source of your eggs or poultry, like purchasing from a local farm. Or choose organic, which is always free-range.

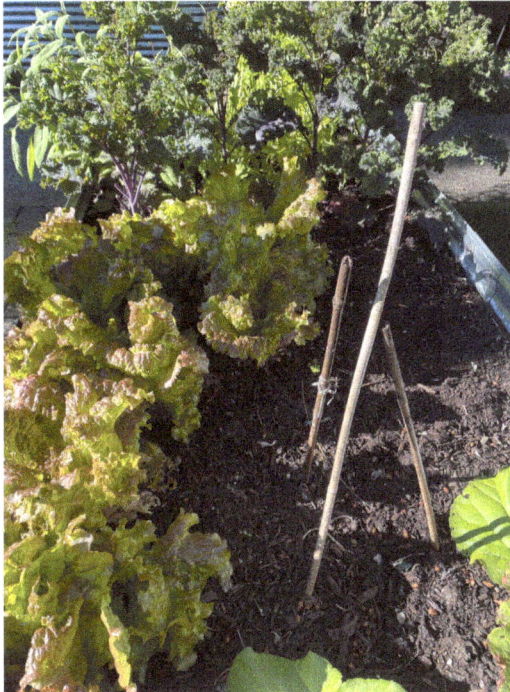

Organic foods are grown without the use of many synthetic chemicals, like pesticides and herbicides. Organic farming also bans the use of genetically-modified organisms (GMOs), which are often highly linked to extensive use of agro-chemicals and deny farmers the basic right of seed-saving due to the patenting of life. Organic farming is all about soil and environmental health, so practices like crop rotation are important as well as protecting pollinator species like bees and butterflies.

Organic certification can be expensive for small farmers, so try to know more about the source of your foods and whether farmers may employ organic practices, like limiting agro-chemicals, but have not gone through the laborious and expensive process of certifying their farm.

Not all organic foods are created equal. Some crops require many more inputs and retain more of the agro-chemicals when they get to your plate. Check the **Resources** section for further information but try to choose organically-grown berries, peaches, cherries, grapes, apples, green beans and leafy greens. On the other hand, there are some crops that naturally require less inputs or retain less chemicals, often fruits and vegetables where we cannot eat the peel, like melons, bananas, avocados, mangos and pineapple so this is where you can choose conventionally grown versions.

Foods that contain fat, like milk and meat, have more potential to retain agro-chemicals as they are stored in fat cells. Prioritize your organic dollars for these foods, if you choose to eat animal products, and although they may cost more, try to consume them less often as plants have much less impact on climate change overall and they are much better for our health.

Eating any food is more important that eating organic food, but if you do have the option, why add to the toxic load on your body, especially during a time of detoxification and recovery? The liver is responsible for detoxifying the body, and it may be damaged from years of heavy substance use. Lighten its load by minimizing the toxins you consume, whether from pesticides or from the preservatives and additives commonly found in ultra processed foods, and feed it well with antioxidants from vegetables and fruit.

Cooking at home is another way to be more sustainable as you can choose which ingredients you buy and limit the amount of packaging you consume. Restaurants and especially fast food establishments are often looking for the most inexpensive ingredients to protect their bottom line. They are rarely concerned with your health or that of our planet. That said, we all enjoy eating out occasionally for convenience or to try something that we don't cook for ourselves. Aim for eating out as a maximum once per week and that includes the stop for a coffee and muffin. Single-use coffee cups are a huge source of garbage as they are rarely recycled properly.

Packaging is another issue for our planetary health. Single-use plastic beverage containers are energy intensive and end up in our oceans with many individuals and nations not recycling properly. Soft plastic bags or overwrap can easily form the bulk of our household garbage but many communities now allow you to separate it for recycling, although sometimes you have to take it to the recycling depot yourself.

At home, avoid plastic wrap and choose reusable containers and beeswax wrap for storing food or packing lunches. Bring your cloth bags when you go grocery shopping and pack your own water bottle and coffee mug when you are going out.

Tips on Sustainability

- Consider the impact of your food choices on our planet
- Eating any food is more important than eating sustainable food
- Learn more about where your food comes from and how it is grown or harvested

Self-Reflection on Sustainability

Food is one of the major causes of climate change. Is there one change you could make to your food choices this week to help the planet (e.g. cooking at home, prioritizing plant-based protein foods)?

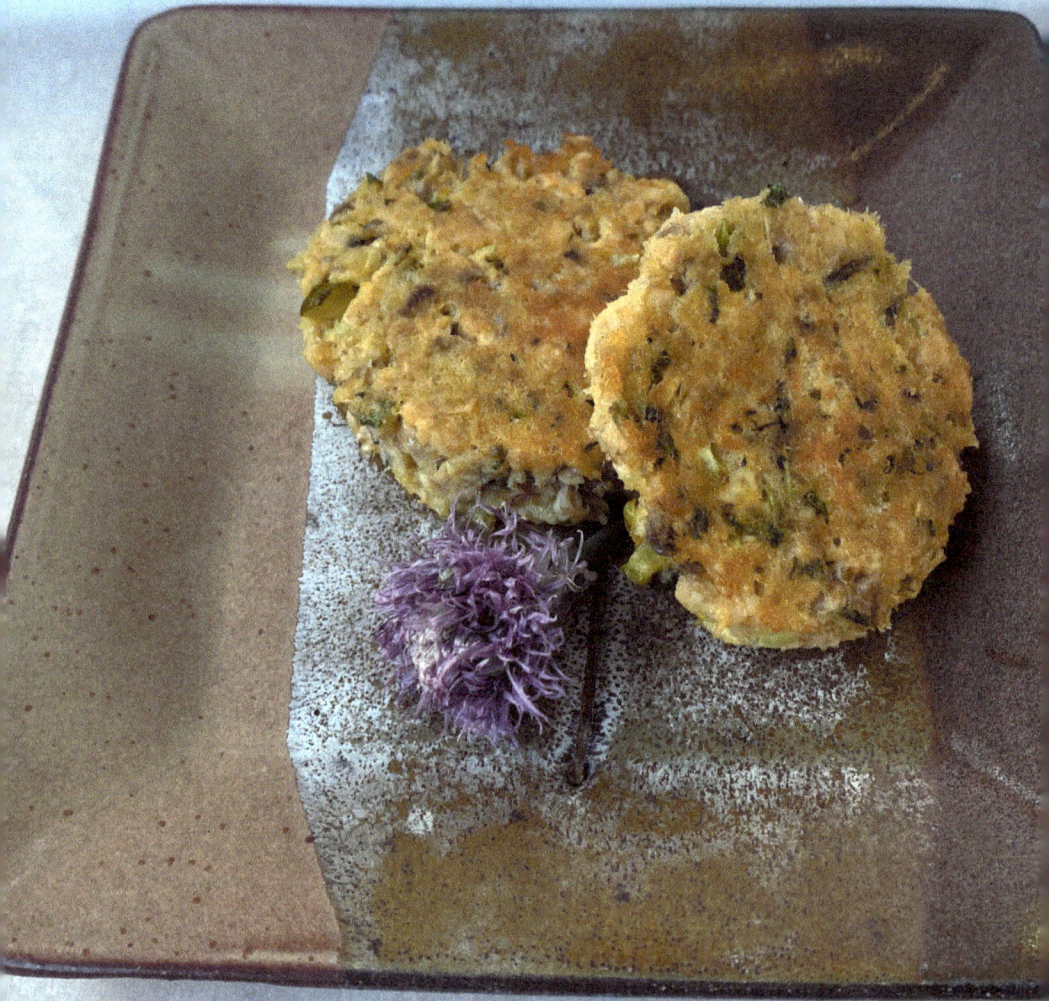

Salmon Cakes

Canned salmon is a perfect pantry staple to make a protein-filled meal come together quickly. Salmon is one of our best sources of essential omega 3 fat and vitamin D.

Serves 4

2 cans wild salmon, preferably with the skin and bones
2 eggs
1 Tbsp mustard

1/2 cup rolled oats, panic or homemade bread crumbs
1/2 cup finely chopped celery, pickles or green onion
2 Tbsp olive oil

In a large bowl, combine salmon, eggs and mustard, mashing well to break up salmon. Add the oats and celery, pickles or onion.

Heat a large skillet on medium low heat then add 1 Tbsp olive oil. Form 1/2 cup of salmon mixture into a patty then place in the pan and repeat, making 3 or 4 more patties. Use a spatula to press the patties down and push around the edges to tuck in any bits that break off. Fry until golden, approximately 3-5 minutes then flip and fry for 3-5 minutes on the other side. Remove to a paper towel-lined plate and keep warm. Repeat with the remaining salmon mixture, adding another 1 Tbsp olive oil to the pan.

Serve with Yogurt Herb Dipping Sauce.

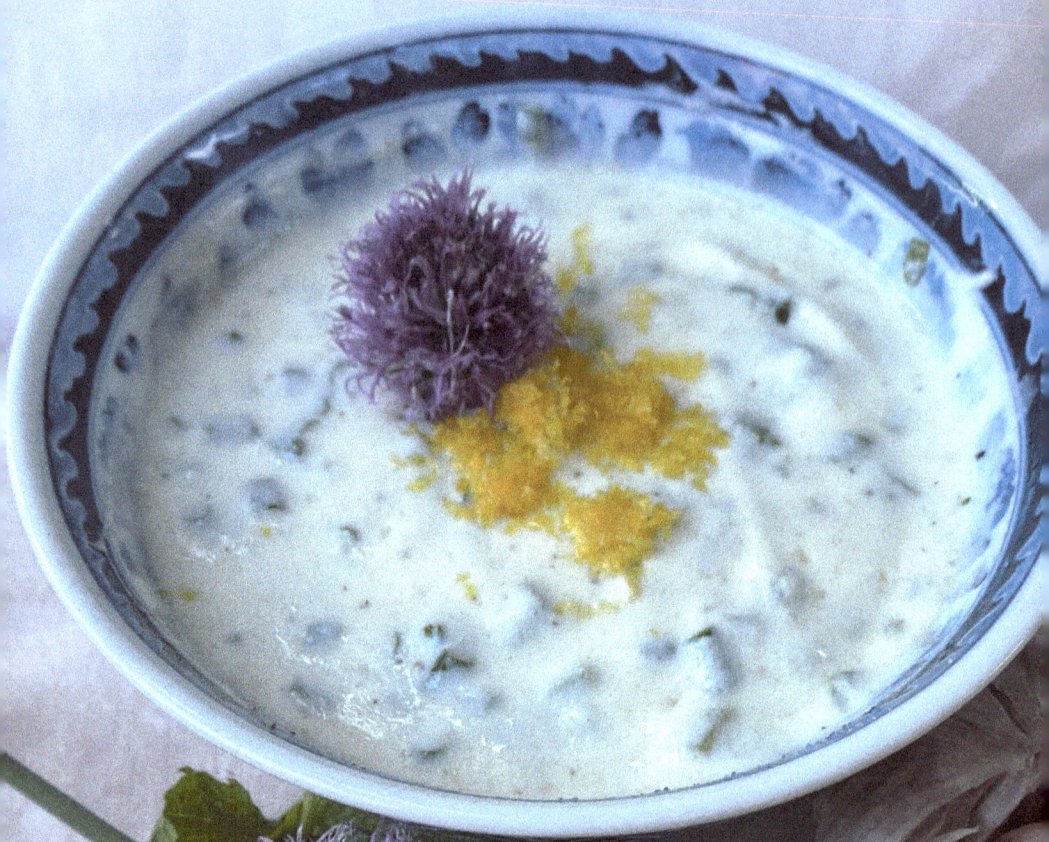

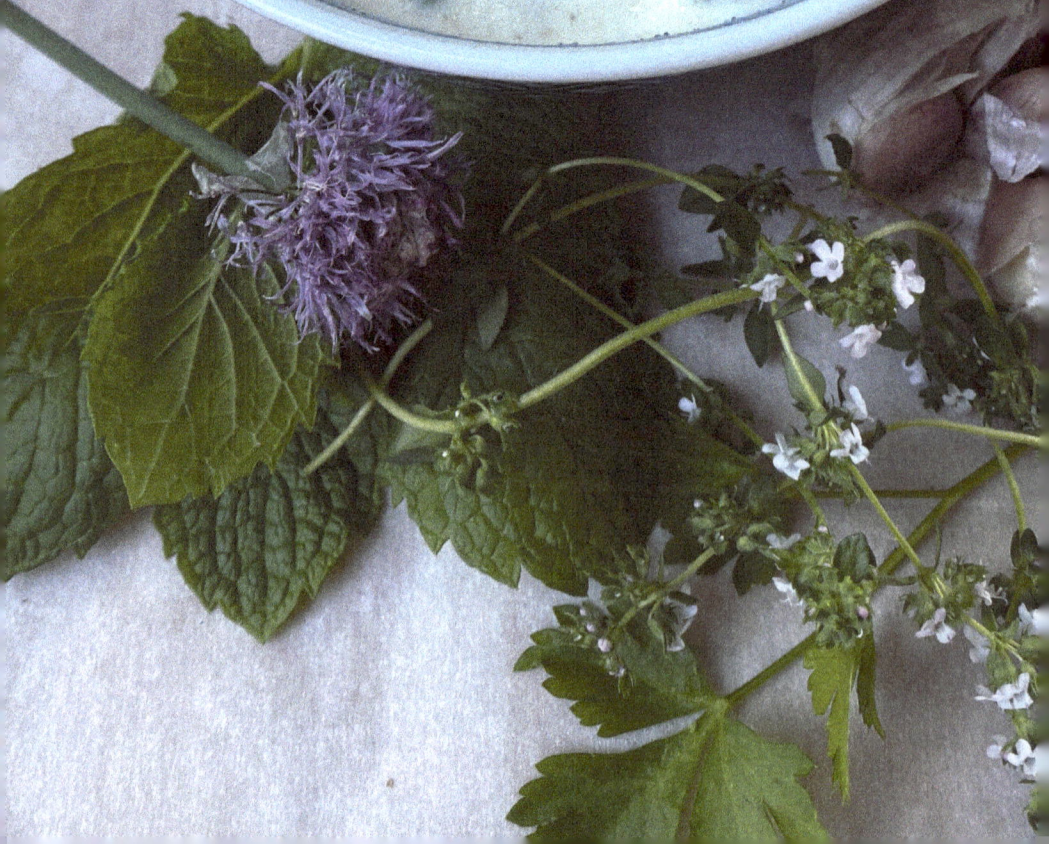

Yogurt Herb Dipping Sauce

This delicious dip or dressing is so easy to make and contains better nutrients than store bought versions. Use with fritters, on salad or serve with raw veggies.

Serves 4

1 cup plain, preferably Greek, yogurt

1 Tbsp olive oil

1/4 cup fresh herbs (e.g basil, dill, parsley), diced

Zest and juice of 1 lemon

1 clove garlic, minced

1/4 tsp salt

Pepper to taste

Simply combine all ingredients in a small bowl or jar. Store leftovers in the refrigerator for up to 1 week.

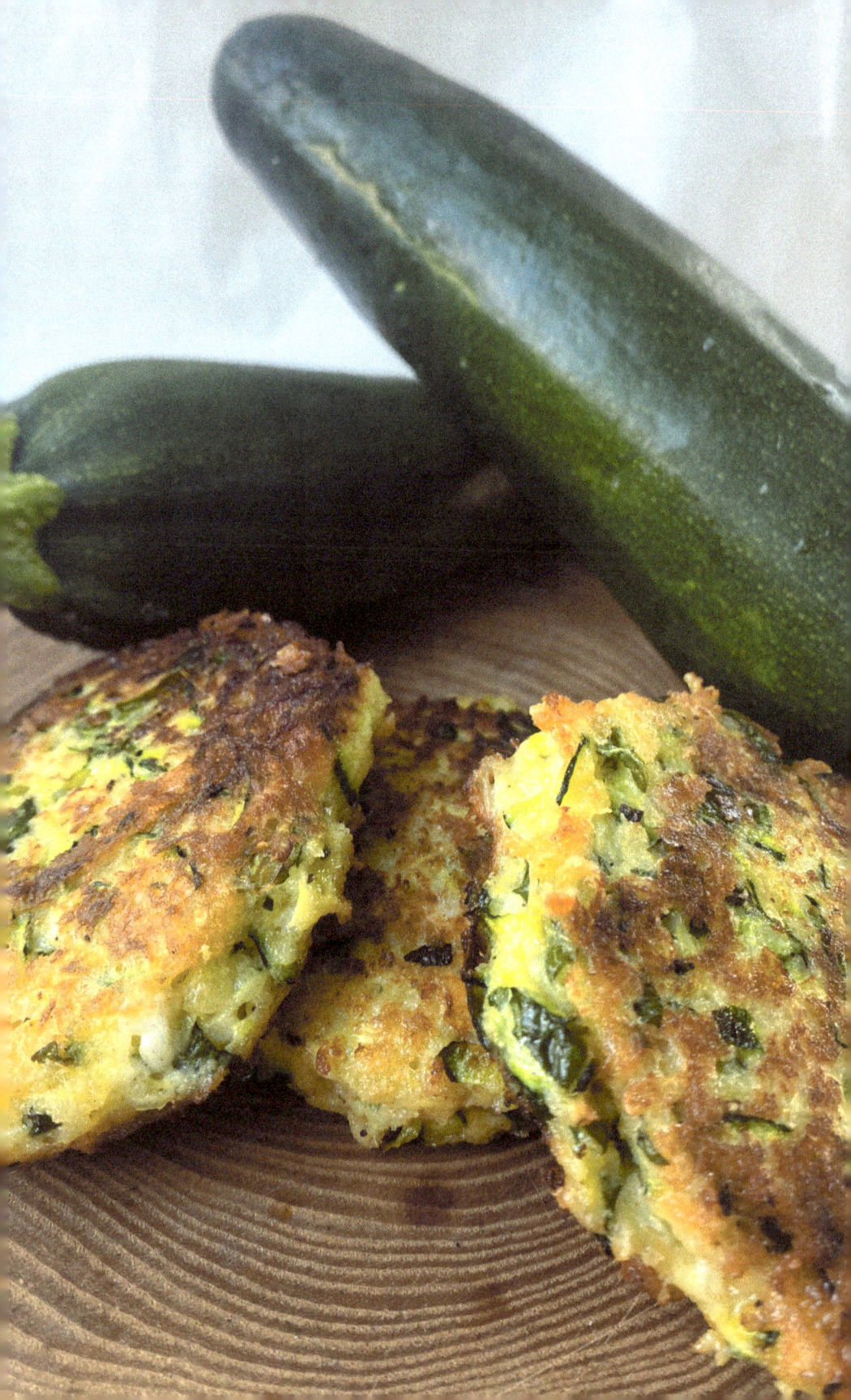

Zucchini Fritters

A great way to use up veggies or cooked grains in a delicious and different way! Simply combine grated or pureed veggies, like zucchini, carrot, pumpkin, squash or potato with grains, rolled oats or homemade bread crumbs and some egg to bind it together.

Serves 4

2 cups zucchini, grated
1/2 tsp salt
1 cup rolled oats, panko or
homemade bread crumbs
2 eggs, beaten

1/4 cup fresh herbs (e.g. dill, basil,
parsley), chopped
Pepper to taste
1/2 cup cheese, crumbled or
grated (optional)
2 Tbsp olive oil

Place grated zucchini and salt in a strainer and allow it to sit for 10-15 minutes then press gently to squeeze out excess liquid. Add into a large mixing bowl and mix well with oats, eggs, herbs, salt, pepper and cheese, if using. Heat a large skillet on medium low heat and add 1 Tbsp oil. Take 1/4 cup of zucchini mixture and form into a pattie, then place in pan. Repeat with 3 or 4 more patties. Cook for 5 minutes until golden then flip and cook on the other side for another 3-5 minutes. Remove from pan to a warm oven and cook remaining patties, adding the other 1 Tbsp oil. Serve warm with Yogurt Dipping Sauce.

Cooking And Meal Planning

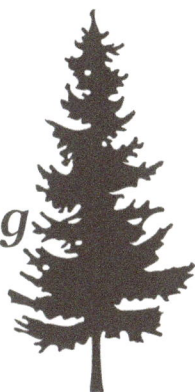

Cooking is a lost art, science and simple way of life for many of us, especially in addiction. Before the days of ultra processed, convenience and fast foods, most people did all of their cooking at home, and they were much healthier for it. Today we rely on foods that do not provide the nutrients we need, especially fibre, vitamins and minerals and instead are abundant in less healthy nutrients like salt, sugar and saturated fat. This has led to the current metabolic crisis in North America and other countries around the world with diabetes, heart disease and cancer deaths skyrocketing.

Cooking though, is more than just understanding what goes into your meals and eating more nutritiously. It connects us to our food, the land (or sea) it came from, honouring those who work so hard to provide these foods for us. It also connects us to our history, culture, traditions, family and friends. Eating together with others has numerous benefits and in areas of the world with the highest longevity, these social practices are key.

When you are living with addiction, acquiring and using your substances, takes up so much space in your life, it doesn't leave much time for food. Addiction displaces your appetite, drains your budget, and the love of good food is lost. You no longer get the light dopamine lift from eating good food as the dopamine pathway in your brain has been altered.

So when we don't get the normal pleasure of eating that we should, it definitely decreases any desire to cook. Or in acute addiction, we may be unable to cook, we may have lost access to kitchens and groceries. And what food we do take in, just to eke out a bare existence, may come from ultra-processed convenience foods, corner stores, fast food establishments and for some, shelters and food banks. These latter important food security resources can provide more nourishing food but it's not always a guarantee, as they are often dependent on what food they receive.

Getting started cooking does not have to involve elaborate chef-style meals as we see on food shows. In fact, we don't even have to use the term cooking if that's intimidating for you. Let's just call it home food preparation and likely you have done some of it before, like making a piece of toast or frying up an egg, assembling a sandwich or putting together a salad. These are the starting points and they are much preferred to eating out, usually much more affordable and they also have the ability to contain more nutrients.

Souping it up is the next step, which is my term (borrowed from the car world!) for taking a convenience food and making it more nutritious. For example, using a canned or packaged soup but adding extra vegetables, cooked whole grains or beans, peas or lentils to boost the fibre, vitamins and minerals and balance out the excess sodium. Other examples of souping it up, would be to use a packaged dough and make your own pizza, biscuits or bread, adding extra vegetables, cheese, nuts and seeds.

Rotisserie chicken, from the grocery store, is another great starting point. They are often "loss leaders", meaning grocers make very little money on them as a way to get you in the store to spend money on items that they do make margin on, like ultra-processed foods. Rotisserie chickens are not much different, nutrient wise, from making your own roast chicken. Use them first for a simple meal of chicken, whole grains or potatoes and veggies. Then pull off the extra meat and store it in a sealed container in the refrigerator, to use for sandwiches, wraps, salads, tacos, quesadillas, stir fries or grain bowls. The bones can be stored in a sealed bag and used to make *Simple Chicken Soup*, which you'll find in the recipe section.

Moving on to the next step in home cooking is to use simply processed foods like dry pasta, canned legumes, fish or vegetables, to make easy, nutritious meals come together quickly. Stock up regularly on these pantry staples, which are often also available at food banks and corner stores, and are very affordable.

Traditional family recipes might be the next step, connecting us to our culture and wonderful food memories with our families. Learning from our elders keeps these traditions alive and helps recognize the wisdom these family members hold. My maternal grandfather, Poppa, was an avid cook. His specialty was making soup and he was passionate about minimizing food waste. He saved all the bones from meat dishes and used up all the vegetables that were ripening too quickly. His Potato Soup is the lore that my family dishes upon and it fills us with special memories of sitting around his table.

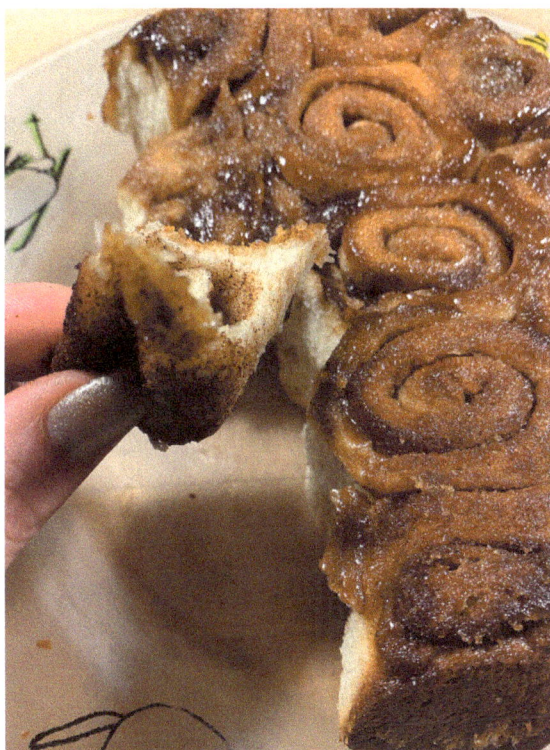

My maternal grandmother, Nanny, was an avid baker and her grandchildren always helped in the kitchen making her signature Cinnamon Buns, Oatmeal Cookies, Rhubarb Raspberry Crisp and Perogies. Just the smell of these foods baking brings tears of joy to my eyes and connects me to her and the comfort she gave.

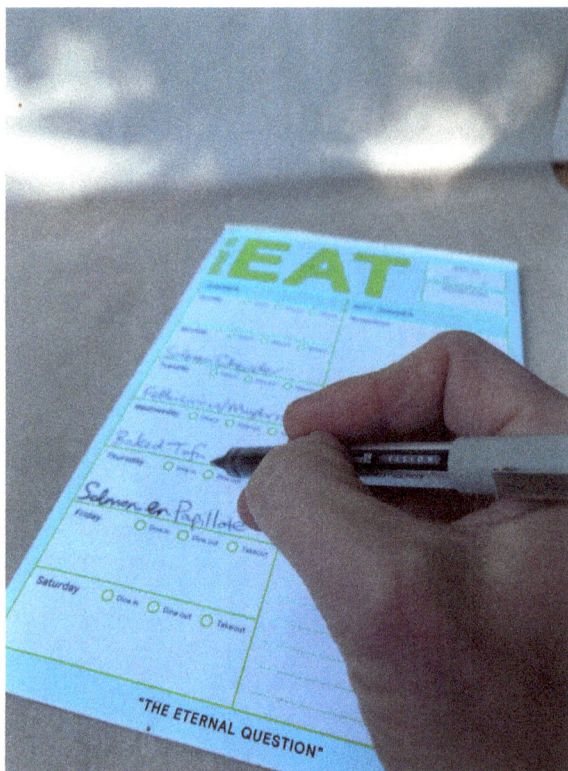

"THE ETERNAL QUESTION"

Meal planning is the key to making meals come together quickly and without the stress that often arises around 5pm when we get off work and have to figure out what to make for dinner. When we are tired and hungry, we often opt for fast, convenience foods rather than take the time to cook at home. But making a meal plan and having the foods available can take this stress away and you may even find the time you spend cooking can be joyful and relaxing.

Check the fridge, freezer and pantry first, when making your meal plan, to determine what you need to use up. Minimizing food waste is not only important for our planet, but it saves so much money that often goes into the compost or garbage. Base meals around vegetables, tofu or animal proteins that need to be used, adding groceries from the store to round out the meal.

Choose from your standards next for easy meals on weeknights and save more elaborate recipes for when you have more time. Eating the same thing each week is not a bad thing and that consistency can be comforting. Perhaps it's a simple pasta dish with chickpeas, spinach and feta cheese. Or tacos filled with refried beans, cheese and veggies.

Grain bowls are another easy weekday meal that can be varied to keep things fresh and to appeal to those with diverse food likes and dislikes, namely children! Cook large batches of whole grains, like brown rice, quinoa or millet, and keep them in the fridge for the base of a bowl. Then choose a protein, whether leftover cooked chicken, canned legumes, baked tofu, sautéed shrimp or canned fish. Add veggies that tie in, perhaps some raw, like bell peppers, cucumbers, avocado or grated carrot, and some cooked like roasted sweet potato, squash, nugget potatoes and onion. Finally add a sauce, like *Miso Tahini* from the chapter on **Digestive Health**, Avocado Crema which is simply made with Greek yogurt, lime juice and mashed avocado or a Spicy Mayonnaise. Fermented condiments like kimchi and sauerkraut can add some delicious flavour and of course the probiotic bacteria that is key to gut health.

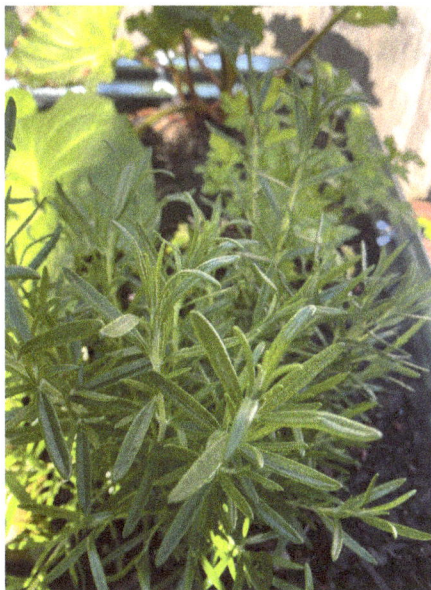

Herbs and spices are the key to delicious food that does not have to be loaded with salt. Fresh herbs are easier to use than spices when you first start cooking. But they can also go bad quickly. One tip is to store them stem side down in a jar of water, with a bag placed loosely over top. Experiment with a new bunch of fresh herbs each week, adding fresh basil or flat-leaf Italian parsley to pastas, cilantro to tacos and coleslaws, fresh dill to eggs or even tearing some herbs up and adding them as a salad green.

Rosemary, thyme and sage are herbs that are easy to grow but are better used in cooked dishes. Add rosemary to marinades for tofu or meat. Use thyme in warm, comfort dishes like stews and soups, fish "en papillote", meaning cooked in pastry or wrapped in parchment, and any dish based on mushrooms. Sage is delicious with tempeh or poultry dishes

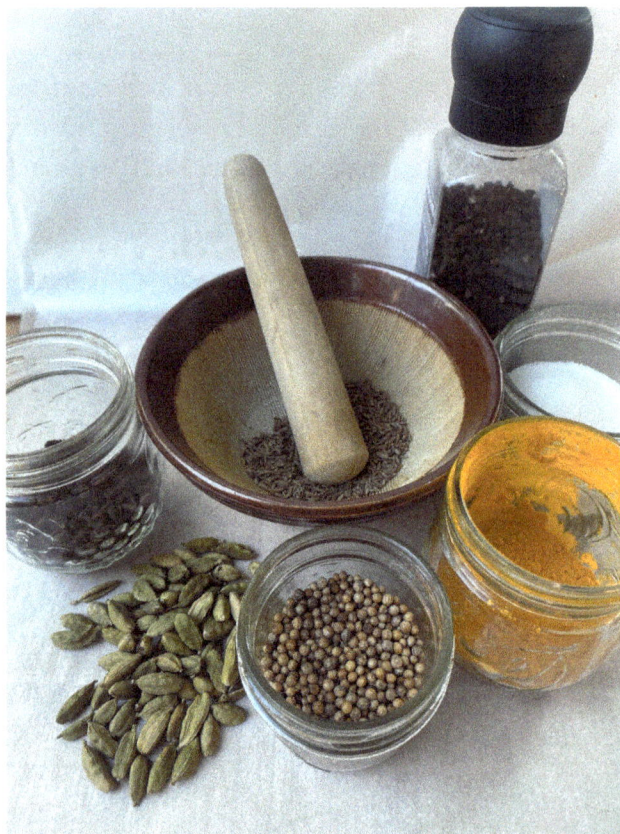

Spices are the next thing to stock in your pantry. Cumin is a common addition to Mexican cuisine like refried beans, as well as in Indian curries, along with turmeric, the signature yellow spice that forms the basis of curry powder. Smoked paprika can be added onto roasted vegetables, in eggs and meat dishes. Italian seasoning or oregano are great for pasta sauces and Pasta Fazool soup. Spices like cinnamon are often used in baking but also as an addition to African savoury stews. Be cautious with cinnamon, nutmeg, cloves and allspice which can easily overpower a dish.

Lemon and lime are also great for using without as much need for added salt to flavour a dish. Use the zest, being careful not to get down to the bitter, white pith, for a blast of flavour in yogurt dips, sauces and baking. Use the juice at the very end of cooking to bring freshness to a curry, stir fry or soup. Lemon or lime juice are also great acidic components of Homemade Salad Dressings and to use in marinades for tofu, fish or poultry.

Onion and garlic form the basis of most cooked cuisines around the world. They are very affordable, flavourful aromatic vegetables and should be a part of your weekly grocery list. Chopped onion, carrot, celery and minced garlic can be sautéed in olive oil to form a mirepoix or soffrito, the foundation of most soups. Some people find chopping onion to be intimidating or tear-provoking. Using very cold onion can help prevent tears. To chop, first cut off the stem and top, then cut in half widthwise and remove the skin. Take one half and place it cut side down on your chopping board. It's easier to chop things that lie flat than something that rolls around. Then take a large, sharp knife and cut approximately five lengthwise strips. Holding the onion with a flat palm on top, cut one large slice widthwise. Now you can chop the third plane and you will end up with even pieces that can be used in any dish.

For garlic, use a press if you are turned off by sticky fingers. Or now, in many grocery stores, you can buy minced garlic in jars and simply scoop into your hot pan. Don't worry if the garlic sprouts a green top—my Poppa always said this was the best part. Just remove the hard root, the papery peel and any brown spots prior to mincing.

Choosing recipes for when you have more time in the kitchen can be a fantastic way to stay inspired, try new flavours and build your food literacy. Aim to try something new each week or two by asking friends for their favourites, learning from your elders, taking a cookbook out from the library or internet searching for an ingredient you may need to use up.

Start slowly when choosing new recipes. Look for those with fewer steps and ingredients, so you are not overwhelmed.

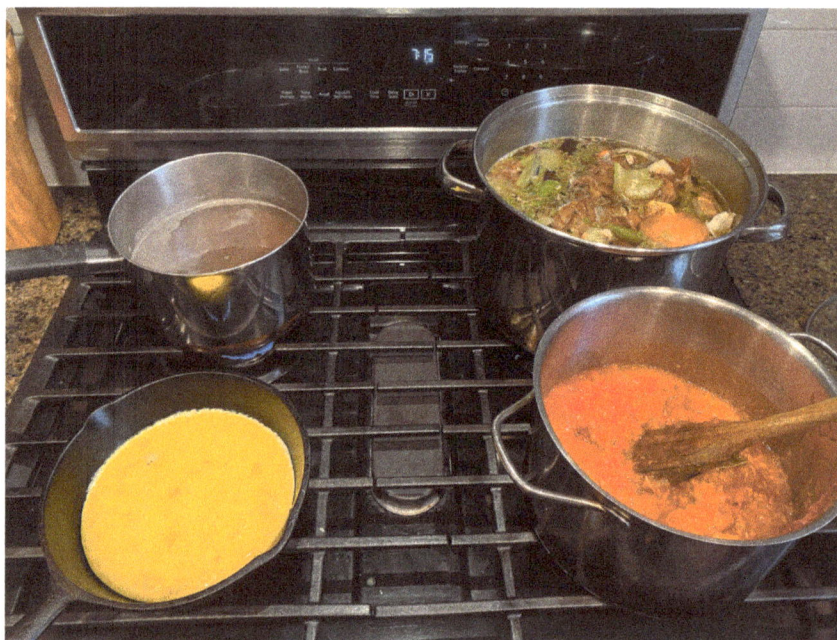

Batch cooking does not have to involve simply making a huge quantity of one dish that you will get tired of eating as leftovers. Consider dishes or simple ingredients that can form the basis of more than one type of meal, like roast chicken or whole grains. Prep extra vegetables for an easy-to-grab snack or to form the basis of a quick weekday meal.

Get together with friends or family to cook together. It's a great, healthy way to socialize in recovery! You can employ the batch cooking method discussed above so that everyone gets to take home an extra dish or two as well as eating one meal together after you've finished cooking. More hands make light work so cooking together might be an opportunity to try a dish that needs an assembly line approach like dumplings, empanadas or perogies.

Tips for Cooking and Meal Planning

- Start slowly—home food preparation does not have to involve elaborate recipes
- Connect with your food culture and traditions
- Make a plan for your meals to use up what you have and shop more efficiently and affordably

Self-Reflection on Your Cooking

Making and eating food together is a central facet of human culture. Is there a food you remember from your childhood that would bring you joy to make? Can you buy one less meal out this week and make one more meal at home?

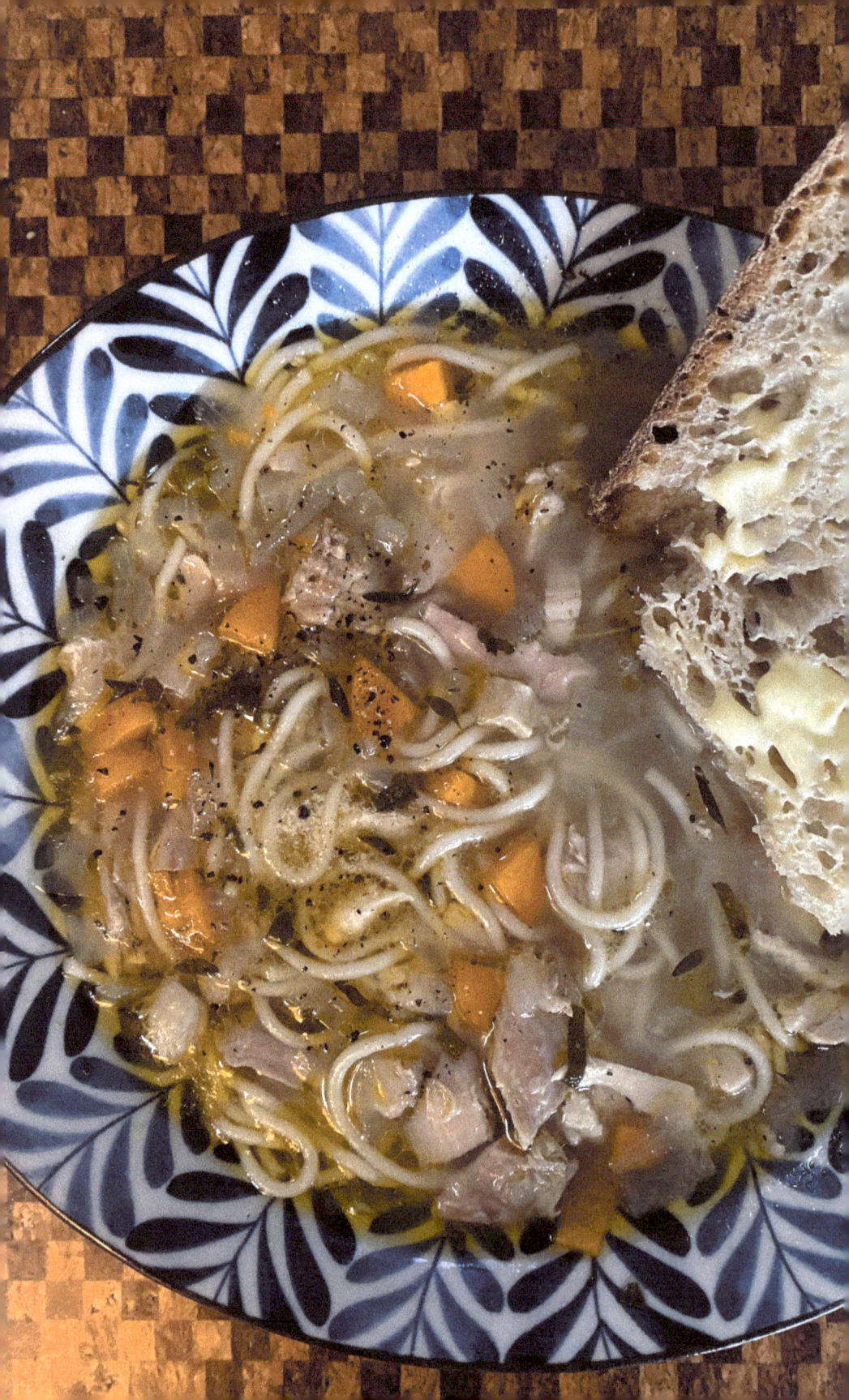

Simple Chicken Soup

Comfort food for the soul, chicken soup often triggers positive memories from childhood, from spending time in the kitchen with family to feeling better when we're sick. This soup is a great way to use up vegetables and create an additional meal from leftover chicken bones, maximizing flavour and nutrients in your soup.

Serves 4

2 Tbsp olive oil
1 onion, diced
2 celery stalks, diced
1 large carrot, diced
3 cloves garlic, minced
2 L chicken or vegetable stock or water
2 bay leaves

Chicken bones (save the carcass from roasted or rotisserie chicken in the freezer)**
Other root vegetables (optional)
2 cups chicken, raw or cooked, chopped
1 cup dry pasta or cooked rice
1 can chickpeas, drained (optional)
Fresh herbs (e.g. parsley, dill), chopped

In a large pot, heat oil on medium low, then add onion, celery, carrot and garlic. Saute for 10 minutes until soft then add stock or water and bay leaves. Bring to a boil. Add chicken bones and return to a boil then reduce heat and simmer for 30 minutes. Remove bones and bay leaves and discard, using a slotted spoon or strainer. Add other veggies and chicken, if raw, then cook for 15 minutes until tender. Add chicken, if using pre-cooked, pasta and chickpeas if using. Cook until pasta is tender, approximately 10-15 minutes. Serve hot garnished with fresh herbs.

**If you don't have bones in the freezer, you can buy bone-in chicken thighs. Brown these first in the olive oil, for about 4 minutes per side, salting liberally, then remove and add the vegetables. Once the veggies are cooked, add the water and return the chicken to the pot. After it is cooked (approx 15 minutes), remove the chicken and allow to cool then remove and discard the skin and bones. Chop the chicken and return to the pot with the pasta.

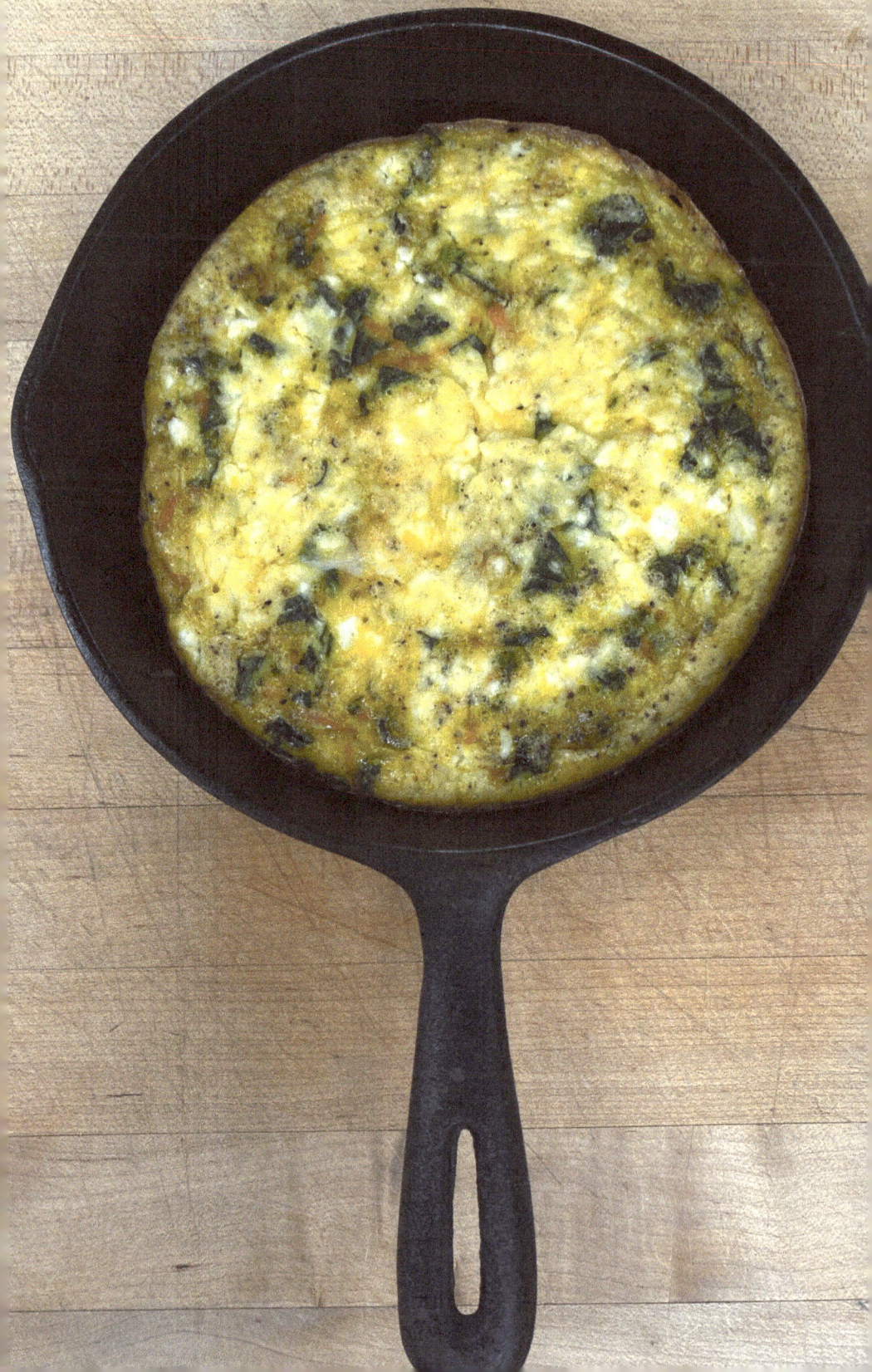

What's in the Fridge Frittata

A quiche without the crust and an easy meal you can make in 15-20 minutes, using up whatever veggies you have in the fridge. For a heartier version, add in some cooked whole grains or potatoes.

Serves 4

1 Tbsp olive oil
1/2 onion or 1 shallot, diced
4 large mushrooms, chopped
2 cups dark leafy greens (e.g. spinach, kale, chard)
1 carrot, grated

10 eggs, beaten
Salt and pepper
1/2 cup cheese, grated or crumbled
1/4 cup fresh herbs (e.g. dill, basil, parsley), chopped

Preheat oven to 350F. In a large, oven-safe skillet, heat oil on medium low then add onion. Saute until onion is soft and golden then add the mushrooms. Saute another 5 minutes then add the greens and cook until wilted. Add the grated carrot then the eggs, ensuring they spread evenly through the pan. Season with salt and pepper then sprinkle with cheese and herbs. Place in the oven and bake for approximately 10 minutes until set and puffed slightly. Serve warm with whole grain bread and/or salad. Refrigerate leftovers for up to 3 days and use as a delicious sandwich filling.

Weekly Meal Plan & Grocery List

As mentioned in the chapter above, taking some time on the weekend to look in the fridge and freezer, consult some recipes (like in this book!) then making a meal plan and grocery list and shopping for the food you need will help to take the stress out of cooking and eating. Here is a sample weekly menu, with suggestions for when to make food in advance to save you time during the week:

Sunday

Breakfast: *Carrot Walnut Muffins** with Fruit, Yogurt and Hemp Hearts

Make ahead: *Chia Pudding* (make this while the muffins bake)

> *freeze leftover muffins for the week

Lunch: Cheese & Whole Grain Crackers with Cucumber & Avocado Slices

Dinner: Roasted (or Rotisserie) Chicken* & Roasted Potatoes and Veggies

> *to roast the chicken, marinate for one hour in olive oil, lemon juice and salt then bake in a 375F oven until internal temperature reaches 74F. To roast the potatoes and veggies, toss with olive oil, salt and pepper and bake on a sheet pan until caramelized and tender (~30 minutes)

> *save the chicken bones for Monday's dinner, make extra veggies for the week

Make ahead: Cook quinoa for the week

Monday

Breakfast: *Chia Pudding* with Fruit, Yogurt and Hemp Hearts

Lunch: Roasted Vegetable, Quinoa and Feta Salad

Snack ideas for any day: Peanut butter or cheese and apple; handful of nuts

Dinner: *Simple Chicken Soup* with Green Salad* and Whole Grain Bread or Crackers

*make a simple vinaigrette by mixing olive oil and apple cider vinegar 3:1 then adding salt, pepper, maple syrup, mustard and chopped garlic (optional). Store in the fridge for up to 2 weeks.

Tuesday

Breakfast: *Carrot Walnut Muffins* with *Green Smoothie*

Lunch: Leftover *Simple Chicken Soup*

Dinner: *Salmon Cakes** with *Yogurt Herb Dipping Sauce* and cut-up veggies*

*make extra for lunch leftovers, sub leftover quinoa for breadcrumbs if desired

Wednesday

Breakfast: *Chia Pudding* with Fruit, Yogurt and Hemp Hearts

Lunch: Leftover *Salmon Cakes* with *Yogurt Herb Dipping Sauce* and cut-up veggies

Dinner: *What's in the Fridge Frittata* with Green Salad (add leftover quinoa to salad if desired) and Whole Grain Bread

Thursday

Breakfast: Oatmeal or Overnight Oats* with Fruit, Yogurt and Hemp Hearts

*make extra oatmeal or overnight oats for leftovers

Lunch: *Frittata* Sandwich on Whole Grain Bread with cut-up veggies

Dinner: *Chickpea Potato Curry** with Brown Rice

*start the curry prep in the morning when you may have more energy, you can turn it off at any step and let it sit then re-heat

Friday

Breakfast: *Carrot Walnut Muffins* and *Green Smoothie*

Lunch: Leftover *Chickpea Potato Curry* with Brown Rice

Dinner: Take the night off cooking and treat yourself to take-out!

Dessert: *Amy's Chocolate Pudding**

*hard-boil the eggs earlier in the day when you are fixing your breakfast or lunch, keep refrigerated

Saturday

Breakfast: Leftover Oatmeal or Overnight Oats with Fruit, Yogurt and Hemp Hearts

Lunch: Tuna Sandwich on Whole Grain Bread, cut-up veggies (take it on a hike or walk in the park!)

Dinner: *Brown Rice Congee**

*make extra for leftovers

Drinks for the week: aim for 9-12 cups (250 mL) of fluid each day from water (tap, infused or bubbly), herbal tea, milk, moderate half-caf coffee, kombucha, non-alcoholic beverages (if these fit for you) and *Nikki-Ade* (if suffering from vomiting or diarrhea)

Grocery List For This Meal Plan

(check your fridge, freezer and pantry and adjust as needed; although this may seem like a lot, once you have some of the staples, you won't need to buy so much next week)

Veggies & Fruit:

- Nugget potatoes
- Onion, garlic, ginger
- Veggies for roasting—carrots, peppers, mushrooms, etc
- Veggies for eating raw—cucumber, baby carrots, jicama, snap peas
- Lettuce
- Fruit—frozen or fresh (e.g. berries, apples)
- Lemons
- Kale
- Avocado
- Fresh herbs (e.g. basil, mint and/or dill)

Protein Foods:

- Bone-in chicken or rotisserie chicken
- Eggs
- Chia seeds
- Walnuts
- Hemp hearts
- Peanut butter (natural)
- Peanuts
- Feta and/or other cheese
- Canned salmon & tuna
- Canned chickpeas
- Milk (2% cow's or unsweetened soy)

- Plain yogurt, Greek if desired

Whole Grain Foods:

- Whole grain bread (freeze once sliced, toast as needed)
- Whole grain flour (wheat or gluten-free all purpose mix)
- Rolled oats
- Brown Rice (short grain)
- Quinoa
- Noodles

Pantry Staples:

- Canned tomatoes
- Canned coconut milk
- Olive oil
- Sesame oil (keep refrigerated)
- Apple cider vinegar
- Dijon mustard (keep refrigerated)
- Cocoa powder
- Maple syrup (keep refrigerated)
- Baking powder and soda
- Salt and pepper
- Spices for curry, as needed
- Herbal tea
- Other beverages that work for you (keep refrigerated)

Conclusion

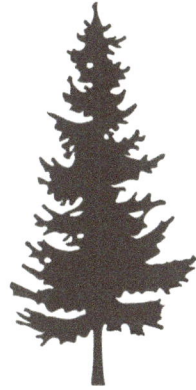

I came home after 4 weeks inspired by my new sober path, eager to put my recovery activities into practice and reconnect with my family and friends. I also knew that for my own recovery, I needed to form a sober community and start planning how to give back. That is what has led to me writing this book as I identified a massive gap in treatment programs on the importance of food and nutrition. I knew my skills, knowledge and experience as a Registered Dietitian along with my personal journey with addiction would allow me to provide a unique perspective that could help others achieve well-being in recovery.

I remained off work for the first two weeks I was back home to give me time to settle in and start a new recovery routine. Luckily I was still part of the Daytox program and they have programming all day, everyday, so I filled my time with 9am Check-In meetings and afternoon acupuncture. I also attended my first Vancouver AA meeting which a Daytox friend had told me about. She was not able to attend, but lucky for me one of my sober lifelong friends came with me for support. The community I feel when I attend an AA meeting is invaluable. Everyone there understands what you are going through in addiction and this is key in recovery, when it can feel like you are alone in your struggles.

Although AA (and its counterparts for other addictions) plays such an important role in our society in terms of providing meetings in almost any place you could go in the world (or online) and at so many times in the week, I struggled with the 12 Steps. I had found my Higher Power in nature, praying to the trees everyday, so Steps 1 and 2 were covered. When I got to Step 3 though, the religious component just would not resonate. I have never been a religious person and I could not wrap my mind around turning over all of my will to my Higher Power. How could the trees be responsible for all of my thoughts, feelings and behaviours?

Instead I have found SMART recovery, which has the same community components and teachings about addiction, yet is free from religion. It also gives autonomy to the individual to have responsibility for their thoughts, feelings and behaviours and this fit much better for me. I attend these meetings weekly, as well as see a psychoanalyst every other week to discuss aspects of my past, present and future that include recovery but so much more.

My husband and I also started back into couples counselling. The trust and intimacy in our relationship had bottomed out when my brother got sick and subsequently died. A wall had formed between us built on his guilt and anger, my self-harm and addictive behaviours, as well as my grief in which I felt completely alone. Fortunately, I have been able to let go of the regret I had carried for years about my brother's suicide and I knew, with work of his own, that my husband could let go of his guilt and anger. He wants to so much as he knows now that my brother's death was also a trauma for him, not just something that happened to me. With time and mutual effort, the wall is crumbling and trust is rebuilding in its place.

Self-care is also a key part of my recovery and overall well-being. I make time to go for a massage or physiotherapy. I meet regularly with my Nurse Practitioner to discuss my medications or get referrals. In acute addiction, there is little time for self-care and health becomes a very low priority compared with getting and using substances.

Exercise is also an essential activity in recovery and life. I dedicate a whole chapter in this book to it as it is extremely beneficial for our physical and mental health. I discovered Barre fitness classes a year ago and have fallen in love with the community and strength I am building there. I go every other day, and often with a friend, which helps in having social activities that are no longer based on substance use. Hiking in the beautiful forests and mountains of North Vancouver are another way to socialize and also enjoy nature and fresh air.

The creativity that I discovered in treatment has also continued at home and I paint regularly (not well!) which I find very meditative. Reading books and writing this one or in my journal are another outlet, especially in the morning when my mind is sharp and I'm drinking my half caf coffee.

Evenings are the toughest time for me. I'm too tired to do anything productive and just feel like watching TV, but I also feel unsettled and restless. That feeling is a trigger for me that used to lead me to drink and smoke a lot of cannabis. Now I find tea is an evening ritual that I look forward to and I like to accompany it with a sweet treat often. I like baking so cookies are often available and I enjoy having a couple to hit the sweet spot.

I've also rediscovered sewing, which is a wonderful activity to keep my hands and mind occupied, especially while watching TV. I have wanted to make a memory quilt for years and have held on to pieces of fabric from old clothing or curtains—they remind me of special times in my life. Crocheting is next on my list to learn, having watched a friend in treatment make a scarf a day and gift one to everyone there.

It is also key for me to eat well. As I have mentioned, I struggle with appetite and I can easily distract my hunger with liquids like coffee or bubbly drinks like kombucha or non-alcoholic beer. But when I am hungry, I feel more anxious and unsettled and eating definitely helps me relax and improve my mood. I still start the day, just like in treatment, with chia pudding topped with berries and hemp hearts or sometimes I will make a smoothie.

Now that I am back to work, I have to consciously take a lunch break, as I have a tendency to want to get everything done before I eat. Leftovers are my go-to but if they have been sent for lunch with my husband or kids, I will make a tuna sandwich or some eggs. Then we always have a nourishing, balanced dinner. I like to have this planned in advance to avoid the stress of thinking about what to make after work. I also like to do some prep in the morning as a break from sitting at my desk and to space apart the meal-making into smaller pieces.

We have some weekly routine meals like bean tacos, mac & cheese, baked tofu & potatoes, grain bowls, soups, shrimp & polenta and then every week or two, throw in a chicken or salmon dinner. If we both have to work late, take-out is an option as we live in an area with so much to choose from. Sushi or pizza are usually the standards and it's a nice change from cooking.

My first party happened after I was home for 5 weeks. A close friend was turning 50 and I was so excited to go and celebrate her with all of our friends. After weeks of being mostly at home, I couldn't wait to get dressed up and put on make up! I felt very strong and confident, eager to show off the new me. I wasn't nervous about the triggers of other people using, despite having committed leaving treatment to not put myself into situations like this one. I knew that I would be content drinking my favourite non-alcoholic wine, eating good food and connecting with others in my new, clear state of mind.

The only thing I was concerned about was the issue that I had been having "using" dreams all week leading up to the party. In one, I was celebrating with a bottle of champagne at a family wedding and I knew I should't be. In another, I threw a giant house party and was extremely repulsed by all the other partiers. In the third, I felt intoxicated and hated the lack of clarity. Most of the time when I have what I call a "stress dream" or in treatment, they call nightmares, I am trying and unable to get somewhere and I am responsible for others, like my children. When I use in these dreams, I lose my sense of control and I believe this is what I ultimately fear.

I shared all of this with my psychoanalyst and we worked through these feelings. She agreed I was processing and preparing for the party and that was very healthy. It wouldn't have been smart to go without planning for such a momentous occasion in my recovery.

The other thing we discussed was my anxiety around my husband at the party. For a couple of years while I was in acute addiction, parties were a sore subject. He would refuse to attend if I was going to be drinking. He would ask me to be the designated driver as a way to attempt to keep me sober, but that rarely worked. Instead I would agree to his terms but drink in secret, alone and obsessing about hiding and sneaking my consumption.

I asked him ahead of the party if we could talk about it and share how he could best support me. Number one was not drinking himself, number two was to be ready to "Batman" out if I felt triggered. But the most important one was to not be supervising me all night. I felt so confident and strong that I didn't want to feel his distrust or worry that I couldn't do it. Of course I have compassion for his feelings around this as I had broken that trust on countless occasions while I was in my addiction.

He agreed to my terms and we had a lovely night. I allowed myself to drink a whole bottle of my favourite non-alcoholic wine, which I usually only drank in smaller amounts because it's not cheap! I ate the delicious food—so much cheese, but balanced by some veggies and hummus and a BBQ tofu sandwich. I wasn't triggered by others drinking but I did feel a little twinge being around cannabis. Not an urge to use really but a longing for the relaxation that I enjoyed when smoking it for decades. The biggest issue was that I was tired by about 9:30pm because that's usually when I go to bed at home.

One of the best parts of the party was sharing with my friends about how amazing I feel. I truly love being sober. I love the clarity. I love feeling joy at the small things in life, like seeing the spring buds coming out on the trees or the sun warming my face. I love my new rituals and routine, like writing at 6am with coffee in the morning before my family wakes up and drinking herbal tea after dinner. I love spending time with my children, snuggling with my boy while I read to him before bed. I love the connection I feel with my daughter lately, despite her natural teenage ability to withdraw, comforting her when she's sad and inspiring her creativity with my own. I enjoy spending time with my husband now, often in the hot tub, when we can share about the work we are doing on ourselves and our relationship, or making plans for all of the trips we want to take together.

I appreciate how fortunate I am that I sought help before I lost all of this support in my life. I met many friends in treatment who haven't been so lucky and I know it is so much harder for them to stay sober when they are facing all the stresses of trying to rebuild their lives. Although I am feeling strong and joyful in my sobriety, I know I have to continue to be vigilant about my recovery. The statistics on relapse are grim and many of those I met in treatment have had to go back for more.

One situation that arose 6 weeks out of treatment was a work trip to Victoria. In my acute addiction, a trip like this meant a bit of a bender, out from under the watchful eyes of my family. Despite systems in place with my husband for me not spending money on alcohol, like cutting up my debit card and denying myself access to cash, I still had a credit card. He could see transactions for liquor stores on our banking app, but I devised many workarounds to get my substance.

One of my tricks was to go to the one grocery store in Victoria that sells wine. This way I could buy it and on the credit card, it would look like I bought groceries. In recovery, I still have this option available to me and it definitely crossed my mind. How would anyone know? But as I learned to do in treatment, I "played the tape forward". If I bought and consumed wine, I knew I would be filled with shame and regret. I would lose my weeks of dedicated sobriety and compromise not only my new "recovery identity" but also put me at risk of a much larger relapse. That certainly didn't seem worth one night of drinking. So I did the right thing even with no one watching.

I also put many other strategies in place for my trip. The first was to make plans, for my time when I wasn't working, that would help to keep me safe and occupied. I organized a lunch date with 3 of my friends from treatment who were in second stage housing in Victoria and I planned to talk to them about my thoughts of using. I also asked a close friend to come and stay with me overnight, to catch up and have fun together, but also because I knew she would keep me on the straight and narrow, having been a huge supporter of my decision to go to, and my time in treatment.

On the morning of my trip, I made sure to eat breakfast. Usually the excitement of a trip and the anxiety around packing and getting out the door on time would put a major curb on my appetite. By getting up with a few hours to get ready, I could be more relaxed and be able to eat. Smoothies are one of the best tools for me in the morning when I am feeling rushed and do not want to sit down and take time to eat.

I also packed supplies for the car, where I knew I could be tempted to pull off the highway at one of the liquor stores I used to frequent. I filled my travel mug with tea and had cold beverages like kombucha and non-alcoholic beer. I packed enjoyable snacks like salted cashews, fresh raspberries (my favourite fruit) and some chips as a treat. All of these foods and drinks bring me joy and take away my urge for booze.

Most importantly I allowed the thoughts about using to come and did not deny them. I acknowledged them and talked myself through them with the plans I had set. I focused on all of the joyful things I had planned and packed. And it worked! However you can never plan for everything that will happen. When I picked up one of my friends from treatment for lunch, I came face to face with a haunting memory from my past. The house where my brother killed himself. It hit me like a ton of bricks—my stomach felt like lead and my heart gaped open. I didn't want to tell my friend what had happened where he was staying, although he knew the story well from our time in treatment together.

We shared a lovely lunch and it was so nice to catch up with my friends, hear how well they were doing in second stage and to reminisce about our time in treatment. After I dropped them off, I burst into tears in the car. I decided to go and visit the spot in the Highlands where we placed some of my brother's ashes. I cried all the way there and even though I didn't have the urge to use, I still called everyone I could, for support, just in case. Then I walked up the hill to his spot, listened to the playlist I made when he died and had a good cry.

The grief will always be there but I don't have to deal with it in the way I used to, by numbing my feelings with substances. I can talk it out with those who love me and him, I can cry and tell him I miss him and I can appreciate the beauty of the spot under the arbutus tree where his ashes lie. When I woke up the next day, I felt one hundred percent better and excited for a new day. I watched the sunrise as I drove to pick up my friends again and go with them to their regular 7am AA meeting. I shared this story and how I was feeling with the group at the meeting. I prayed to the trees with my friends and then drove by the ocean all the way up to work, appreciating its calm endless expanse.

I also find it incredibly important to celebrate my recovery milestones. The first came when I got out of treatment and attended my first Vancouver AA meeting. My best friend got me a lovely cake to celebrate.

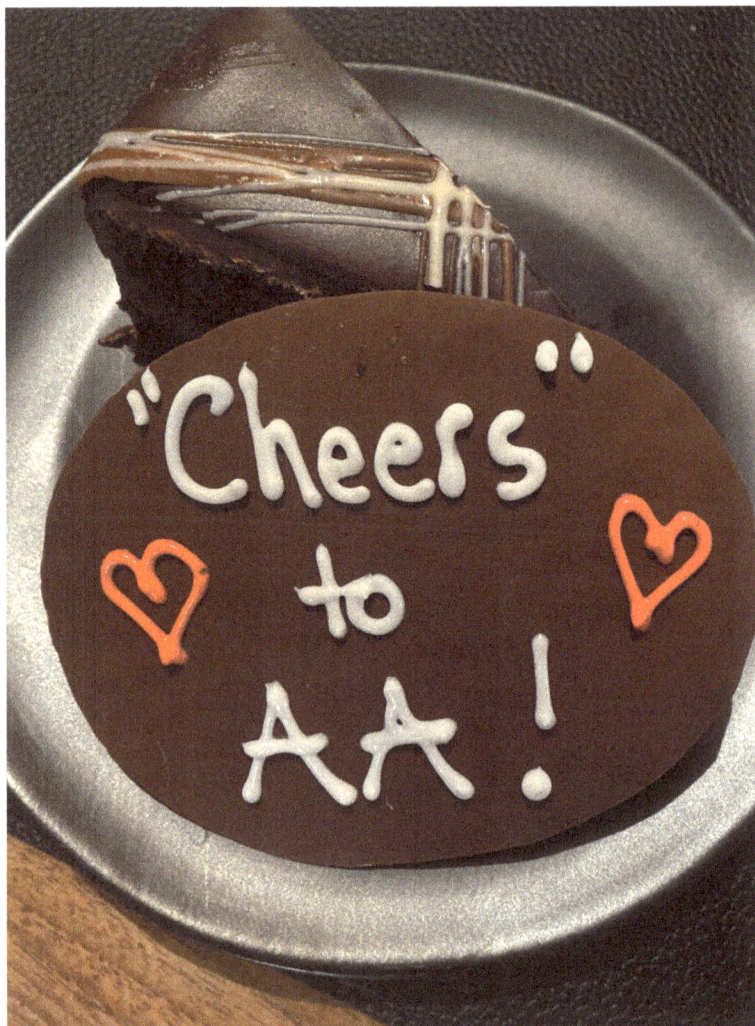

Later that first month out of treatment, I wanted to get a tattoo to symbolize my time there and my new spirituality and path in life. I had been praying to the trees everyday as you can find before the Introduction of this book. So I decided to get a tattoo of a tree with the words "rooted" and "free", because that is how I feel in sobriety. I chose my left bicep because it's close to my heart and every time I flex my strong arms in my Barre classes, I see it and it brings me joy and reminds me of my strength.

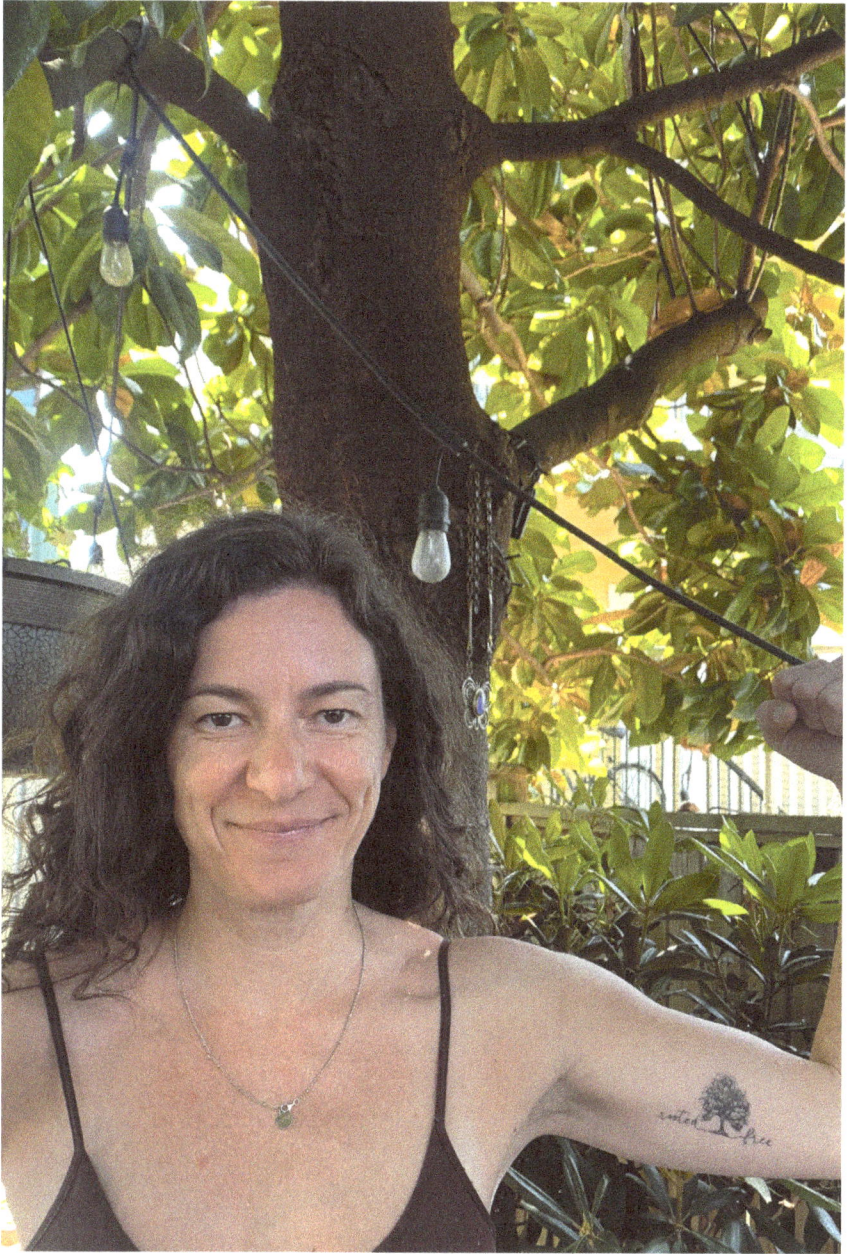

Consider the ways you can celebrate your recovery milestones, whether with cakes, making a new playlist that inspires and speaks to you about who you are now, buying something special for yourself, whether a piece of jewelry, an item of clothing that makes you feel good or maybe a tattoo, like me, or going out with some of your friends from recovery or your family who supports you. The work you are doing is hard and it deserves to be recognized.

Even doing well in recovery, it can still feel shameful to admit you have this disease. You'll never be "normal" the way society makes us feel with alcohol (and now cannabis) being so pervasive. But it's not you that is abnormal, it is the relationship our society has with this toxin, that makes so many of us feel that we cannot celebrate without it.

This book is an attempt to decrease the stigma that I feel and I hope it helps you to lessen the shame that surrounds addiction. In the words of my favourite recovery TV show, Loudermilk, "addiction has taught me compassion, humility and to cherish the small things in life" and I would not have these without the comparative to how bad I felt and how much I lost while deep in my addiction.

Resources And References

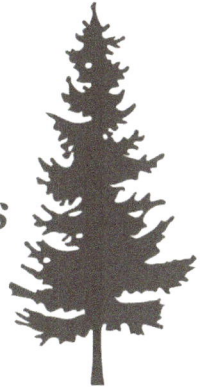

There is a lot of misinformation on the internet about food and nutrition. Try to select information from reputable sources, like those from government, educational institutions and NGOs (non-government organizations). The following are a few you can count on:

The specific nutrient amounts, in food or as supplements, are based on the Canadian and U.S. Recommended Dietary Allowances (RDAs) or Dietary Reference Intakes (DRIs) and can be found here:

> https://www.canada.ca/en/health-canada/services/
> food-nutrition/healthy-eating/dietary-reference-intakes/
> tables/reference-values-elements.html

> https://www.canada.ca/en/health-canada/services/
> food-nutrition/healthy-eating/dietary-reference-intakes/
> tables/reference-values-vitamins.html

For more general information on building a healthy plate:

> Canada's Food Guide: https://food-guide.canada.ca/en/

In British Columbia, HealthLink BC is a free online and phone service where you can access Registered Nurses and Pharmacists 24/7 and Registered Dietitians and Exercise Professionals Mon-Fri, 9-5. Call 8-1-1 or visit www.healthlinkbc.ca

To find support from a reputable nutrition professional:

Dietitians of Canada https://www.dietitians.ca

For more support with addiction and mental health:

Canadian Association for Mental Health https://www.camh.ca

For those dealing with specific health conditions, check out these resources:

Diabetes Canada https://www.diabetes.ca

Heart and Stroke Canada https://www.heartandstroke.ca

Osteoporosis Canada https://osteoporosis.ca

Canadian Digestive Health Foundation https://cdhf.ca/en/digestive-conditions/irritable-bowel-syndrome-ibs/

Food Allergy Canada https://foodallergycanada.ca

For those looking for more information on sustainable food choices:

Environmental Working Group

https://www.ewg.org/foodnews/clean-fifteen.php

https://www.ewg.org/foodnews/dirty-dozen.php

Ocean Wise https://ocean.org

Acknowledgements

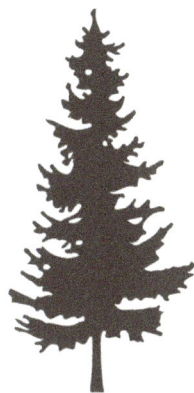

I have learned that it takes a village to publish a book and it's so much more than putting thoughts down on paper. I wish to thank my family of cheerleaders and copyeditors, my Dad, my stepmother Michelle and my sister-cousin Carley for all of their detailed insights. My talented husband Paul, for initiating the inspiring cover design and all of my friends who gave their thoughtful suggestions. Kaitlynn and the team at Friesen Press for holding my hand through this exciting process and providing such valuable guidance. And finally, all my loved ones who supported me in my addiction and recovery, especially the staff at The Healing Institute and the lifelong friends I made there, who shared so much of themselves with me. I couldn't have done any of this without all of you!

Milton Keynes UK
Ingram Content Group UK Ltd.
UKHW050845051224
3429UKWH00037B/151